Communicating With, About, and Through Self-Harm

Lexington Studies in Health Communication

Series Editors: Leandra H. Hernández and Kari Nixon

National and international governments have recognized the importance of widespread, timely, and effective health communication, as research shows that accurate, patient-centered, and culturally competent health communication can improve patient and community health care outcomes. This interdisciplinary series examines the role of health communication in society and is receptive to manuscripts and edited volumes that use a variety of theoretical, methodological, interdisciplinary, and intersectional approaches. We invite contributions on a variety of health communication topics including but not limited to health communication in a digital age; race, gender, ethnicity, class, physical abilities, and health communication; critical approaches to health communication; feminisms and health communication; LGBTQIA health; interpersonal health communication perspectives; rhetorical approaches to health communication; organizational approaches to health communication; health campaigns, media effects, and health communication; multicultural approaches to health communication; and international health communication. This series is open to contributions from scholars representing communication, women's and gender studies, public health, health education, discursive analyses of medical rhetoric, and other disciplines whose work interrogates and explores these topics. Successful proposals will be accessible to an interdisciplinary audience, advance our understanding of contemporary approaches to health communication, and enrich our conversations about the importance of health communication in today's health landscape.

Recent Titles in This Series
Communicating With, About, and Through Self-Harm: Scarred Discourse
    By Warren J. Bareiss
The Ethos of Black Motherhood in America: Only White Women Get Pregnant
    By Kimberly C. Harper
Medical Humanism, Chronic Illness, and the Body in Pain: An Ecology of Wholeness
    By Vinita Agarwal

Communicating With, About, and Through Self-Harm

Scarred Discourse

Edited by
Warren J. Bareiss

LEXINGTON BOOKS
Lanham • Boulder • New York • London

Published by Lexington Books
An imprint of The Rowman & Littlefield Publishing Group, Inc.
4501 Forbes Boulevard, Suite 200, Lanham, Maryland 20706
www.rowman.com

6 Tinworth Street, London SE11 5AL, United Kingdom

Copyright © 2021 by The Rowman and Littlefield Publishing Group, Inc.

Chapter 3 was originally published as Jill M. Hooley, Kathryn R. Fox, Shirley B. Wang, and Anita N. D. Kwashie, "Novel Online Daily Diary Interventions for Nonsuicidal Self-Injury: A Randomized Controlled Trial," BMC Pscychiatry 18, 264, (2018). Reprinted with permission. http://creativecommons.org/licenses/by/4.0/.

Chapter 4 was originally published as Taru Tschan, Janine Lüdtke, Marc Schmid, and Tina in Albon, "Sibling Relationships of Female Adolescents with Nonsuicidal Self-Injury Disorder in Comparison to a Clinical and a Nonclinical Control Group," Child and Adolescent Psychiatry and Mental Health 13, no. [15], (2019): 1–13. Reprinted with permission.

All rights reserved. No part of this book may be reproduced in any form or by any electronic or mechanical means, including information storage and retrieval systems, without written permission from the publisher, except by a reviewer who may quote passages in a review.

British Library Cataloguing in Publication Information Available

Library of Congress Cataloging-in-Publication Data

Library of Congress Control Number: 2020946397

ISBN 978-1-4985-6305-5 (cloth)
ISBN 978-1-4985-6307-9 (pbk)
ISBN 978-1-4985-6306-2 (electronic)

This book is dedicated to people who self-injure. There are reasons for everything, times for making connections, and times for letting go.

This book is also dedicated to Lizah and Ben whose encouragement keeps me moving forward.

Contents

Acknowledgments		ix
Prologue		xi
1	Non-Suicidal Self-Injury: Communicating in Chaos *Marta Carvalhal and Nicole S. Parrish*	1
2	Self-Regulatory Communication in the Treatment of Self-Injury: Development and Maintenance of Therapeutic Rapport *John L. Levitt*	17
3	Novel Online Daily Diary Interventions for Non-Suicidal Self-Injury: A Randomized Controlled Trial *Jill M. Hooley, Kathryn R. Fox, Shirley B. Wang, and Anita N. D. Kwashie*	37
4	Sibling Relationships of Female Adolescents with Non-Suicidal Self-Injury Disorder in Comparison to a Clinical and a Nonclinical Control Group *Taru Tschan, Janine Lüdtke, Marc Schmid, and Tina In-Albon*	57
5	Using Micro-Longitudinal Methods to Examine Social-Communicative Functions of Self-injury in Everyday Life *Brianna J. Turner and Carolyn E. Helps*	83
6	Discursive Tensions and Contradictions: A Cultural Analysis of an Online Self-Harm Forum *Mike Alvarez*	113

7	"Can Airport Scanners See Scars?" An Interpretive Analysis of Self-Injury Narratives *Warren J. Bareiss*	135
8	Fighting the Self: Interpersonal and Intrapersonal Communicative Violence in Chuck Palahniuk's *Fight Club* *Lisann Anders*	161
9	A Systematic Review of Media Use and Non-Suicidal Self-Injury Behaviors *Shuang Liu and Yanni Ma*	183
10	The End (a.k.a The Beginning): Application of Buddhist Principles in *Communicating With, About, and Through Self-Harm* *Warren J. Bareiss*	193

Index	205
About the Authors	209

Acknowledgments

This book would not have been possible without help from many people. First, thanks to Nicolette Amstutz and Sydney Wedbush at Lexington Books and to Daniel Andrew at Deanta Publishing for their generous patience. I am also grateful to John Levitt, Brianna Turner, Carolyn Helps, Mike Alvarez, and Lisann Anders for their encouraging and thoughtful responses to my editorial suggestions in their chapters. Thanks to Jörg Fegert, editor of *Child and Adolescent Psychiatry and Mental Health*, for allowing me to reprint a chapter from that journal and to Taru Tschan who quickly organized all the required paperwork to make that happen. Jill Hooley collected documents needed to reprint a chapter that she cowrote and was readily available to offer advice along the way. My graduate student assistant, Brittany Sterling, proofread new content with a critical and insightful eye for which I am very grateful.

Prologue

Self-injury, self-harm, self-mutilation, non-suicidal self-injury (NSSI)—these terms, and others like them, have been used interchangeably for over twenty years. The fact that the same sorts of behavior go by different names suggests that the topic is still not well understood and is, thus, unpredictable and open to a range of interpretations. Indeed, forms of these behaviors also range widely. Cutting, burning, scratching, banging, and more extreme behaviors such as auto-amputation are conducted under many circumstances by all kinds of people.

This book brings together more than a dozen scholars and clinicians who begin with the same basic starting point but move in directions pertaining to their own specialties. All of the writers here work within the perspective that NSSI is the deliberate harming of one's body without suicidal intent. NSSI is not socially sanctioned, so it does not include such behaviors as tattooing or ritualized scarification. It is typically used as a means of relieving unpleasant emotional states. Possibly due to portrayals in mass media, NSSI is associated in the popular imagination with adolescents, particularly adolescent girls; however, NSSI occurs roughly equally among males and females well into adulthood.

If we know anything about NSSI, we know that it cannot be examined in isolation. NSSI must be considered in light of contextual conditions, such as family dynamics, as well as possibly associated conditions including, depression, stress, and anger. While there is an increased risk of NSSI among psychiatric patients, that population is not the central focus of this book. Rather, chapters in this book address NSSI as the dominant condition in question, albeit with the awareness and recognition that other mental-health related conditions can also be involved.

We have yet to develop a strong understanding of the relationships between NSSI and one of the most fundamental and essential human traits: communication. It is through communication that we not only understand what is happening around us, but also who we are as individuals and as social groups. Is NSSI a form of communication? If so, who is communicating with whom and what are the messages? Also, how is NSSI spoken about by those who engage in self-harm? What are some ways in which clinicians can effectively communicate with patients who self-harm? How is NSSI represented for mass consumption in popular media?

By "communication," I mean the process by which an idea is encoded into a message in the mind of the sender(s), sent through a channel (a medium), and decoded in the mind of the receiver(s). Response from receiver back to sender creates a feedback loop, and this entire process is conditioned by contextual factors including identities of participants, place, politics, culture, economics, and history. Further, noise within the process—a breakdown in communication technology, inability to hear clearly, personal and social biases, confusion on the part of senders and receivers, and so forth—often leads to misperception and misunderstanding. Meaning is never fixed in communication, but rather, is fluid and malleable as messages are encoded and decoded through imperfect, circular, noise-ridden processes. Finally, I would be remiss not to mention that communication continually occurs within our individual minds, leading to the question of how those who self-injure communicate with *themselves* about and through NSSI.

Consider the ways in which communication is evoked in this explanation provided to me by a university student:

> People usually find out by noticing the cuts or scars. I don't usually have formal, sit-down conversations with people about it unless I'm just really struggling and need to talk to someone I trust about it, but if someone that I know respectfully asks about it, I'll answer them. I don't answer random strangers that ask me about it. I just say, "It's personal," and change topics ... I spent years trying to make sure my cuts and scars were always covered, but I don't anymore. I decided that it was nobody's business but my own, and that I shouldn't have to make myself uncomfortable wearing long sleeves or pants when I don't want to just for the sake of making everyone around me comfortable. While my parents are very supportive and understanding of my struggle now, when they initially found out that I was cutting back when I was 13 years old, they were mad, and they grounded me for it. My parents and I have a great relationship, and I don't hold any resentment towards them over it. This was new territory for them, and they didn't know what to do. My friends and coworkers throughout the years have been mostly supportive as well. I suppose I've gotten lucky in that I've always had a pretty solid support

system and people that I can be open about this with. I've known others that weren't as lucky.

This description is an excerpt from an interview that I collected and that the student subsequently edited to get the words just right. Here, we can see communication at the interpersonal level, with the student carefully selecting her words to most accurately represent her circumstances—and I suspect, to also fairly represent herself as an example of the wider population of people who self-injure. The student also mentions further interpersonal communication with her parents, friends, and coworkers—each different types of communication partners with their own sets of expectations, worries, fears, hopes, and so on. Intrapersonal communication is also evident in the student's description of her decision-making process.

In that single passage, the student evokes a richness of detail regarding what it means to self-injure and about the risks of communicating with others about it. At first, the student was unwilling to let me use any part of her transcript in this book, and I can understand why. First, my interview with her did not go well. I was nervous and fearful of saying the wrong thing, given the stigma associated with NSSI. In communicating with the student during the interview, through my verbal and nonverbal communication, I showed myself to be less than confident in my handling of the topic. Even worse, perhaps, once out of her hands, the transcript became *my* message for *my* book, and the student lost control of her words, her message, and her meaning—in a word, construction of herself.

A year passed, and as I was preparing to write this introduction, I reached out to the student one more time. I mentioned how the book was nearing completion and asked if I could use just one or two passages from the interview. This time, with much editing, the student felt comfortable with the passage above.

My engagement with this student provided an important lesson: *How* NSSI is communicated about is as important as *what* is communicated. As such, first and foremost, this book is respectful of people who self-injure and of their circumstances. The purpose of the book is never to judge, but rather, to better understand NSSI, using conceptual and methodological tools available to each chapter writer, ultimately as a service to those who self-injure. Some chapter writers are communication experts, while others are healthcare providers. From our different vantage points, our hope is to broaden understanding of relationships between communication and NSSI so that people who self-injure can be better understood by themselves, by their healthcare providers, and by society at large.

As a communication teacher and researcher, when writing for publication or speaking in public, my first question is generally not about what my message is. My first question is "To whom am I speaking?" Chapter writers sometimes asked me a similar question: Who is the audience for this book? That is the question that I came back to again and again as I collected and edited chapters. Taking my cue from the International Society for the Study of Self-Injury (ISSS), I asked authors to write their chapters in ways that bridge interests and needs of multiple audiences who share a common goal of improving the lives of people who self-injure as well as the lives of those around them. Such audiences begin with those who self-injure, extending to family, friends, teachers, coworkers, social service providers, researchers, and many others in the healthcare industries.

Many perspectives are, therefore, represented in these pages, coming from different places in the scholarly and medical spectrum. Some chapters are qualitative in nature, demonstrating illustrative cases and exploring how individuals and small groups perceive and engage with NSSI on a day-to-day basis. Others are more quantitative in their approach, analyzing large samples through complex mathematical measures. As an editor, I welcome them all. A topic as complicated as NSSI deserves a thorough discussion informed by a diversity of perspectives. I also challenge you, the reader, to try to find something that you can use in each chapter.

We begin with Marta Carvalhal's and Nicole Parrish's discussion of how they work with patients who self-injure day to day in a hospital setting. Carvalhal and Parrish provide a good starting point in laying out an extended discussion of the definition and functions of NSSI. Having created the basic groundwork, they use examples (sans personal identifiers, of course) to demonstrate a range of presenting symptoms and the authors' method of teaching communication skills to patients through dialectical behavioral therapy.

John Levitt also draws upon his work in a clinical setting in chapter 2, but he takes the discussion in a different direction through application of self-regulatory theory. Recognizing the uncomfortable truth that NSSI behaviors often have protective functions for the individual, Dr. Levitt demonstrates how healthcare providers can help patients redirect their intrapersonal communication toward beneficial self-regulation on the path to recovery.

Intrapersonal communication is further elaborated upon by Jill Hooley, Kathryn Fox, Shirley Wang, and Anita Kwashie whose chapter demonstrates that self-criticism so common among individuals who self-injure can be reduced through daily journaling. Further, they describe how effects of maintaining diaries extended to a reduction in the overall number of NSSI incidences, depression, and suicidal ideation amidst their sample. Even so, Dr. Hooley and her co-authors are guarded in their optimism, noting that desire to discontinue NSSI and likelihood of future NSSI occurrences, depression, and suicidal intentions were unaffected by diary writing even when effects in the present are promising. NSSI behaviors and related symptoms, like facts, are stubborn things.

Taru Tschan, Janine Lüdtke, Marc Schmid, and Tina In-Albon shift the focus to interpersonal communication, in this case, among adolescents who self-injure and their siblings. Patterns pertaining to conflict, empathy, coercion, warmth, and other factors among siblings with and without NSSI tendencies lead the authors toward concrete recommendations about coping strategies designed to improve family well-being.

Interpersonal communicative functions of NSSI are further explored by Brianna Turner and Carolyn Helps who describe the socio-communicative functions of NSSI through an extensive review of relevant scholarship. From there, they delve into micro-longitudinal analyses regarding precursors and consequences of NSSI behaviors with respect to socio-communicative functioning and intrapersonal motivations. Here again, personal diaries play an important role—not to reduce incidences of NSSI, but rather, to better understand factors leading to NSSI incidents and their immediate results. Turner and Helps conclude with suggestions for further micro-longitudinal research to better understand the intrapersonal and interpersonal communicative purposes and consequences of NSSI.

Mike Alvarez widens the frame of reference to communication about NSSI among social media users. With this chapter, we move from family and close friends to the "imagined community" (Anderson 1983) of individuals who self-injure. Dr. Alvarez reframes NSSI from a diagnostic position to a cultural descriptor. Using cultural discourse analysis, he examines over 200 messages posted on SuicideForum.com, a website focusing on suicide and NSSI, with a particular focus on emotional precipitants to NSSI behaviors. Significantly, Dr. Alvarez's chapter is the first in the book where we delve deeply into what individuals who self-injure say about themselves, their relationships with others, their motivations, and many other salient factors. As Alvarez notes, stigma associated with NSSI can make talking openly about NSSI difficult, but the anonymity of social media allows those who self-injure to express their attitudes, beliefs, values, and behaviors without fear of retribution.

My chapter similarly approaches discursive style as I explore stories told by and about people who self-injure via a Reddit forum called "r/selfharm." Using Arthur Frank's (1995/2013) illness narrative model, I am particularly interested in what self-injury stories tell us about relationships between the self (i.e., the storyteller) and the body. Like Dr. Alvarez, I found that social media offer valuable insight into the ways that people who self-injure perceive themselves and others, and I would add that the community-based function of social media shifts the style of storytelling away from what one might expect to hear in clinical settings.

Lisann Anders' chapter further explores relationships among NSSI, imaginary community, and media in her analysis of the novel, *Fight Club*. Here, the narrative of self-injury is one of representation and allegory. Deliberate violence inflicted on one's body via participation in a fictional community is a metaphoric reference to loneliness and the desperate need for meaningful interpersonal connection. While the novel is a work of fiction, Dr. Anders continually threads the proverbial needle by linking dominant themes of social angst dramatized in the book to parallel themes of alienation prominently mentioned in NSSI scholarship. Popular culture sometimes reflects and reveals what is hidden in plain sight.

Shuang Liu and Yanni Ma brings the discussion full circle. Beginning with a brief overview of media representations of NSSI, Liu and Ma discuss a wide range of scholarship, arguing that media, in large part, condition how society perceives all kinds of issues, including those pertaining to health and stigma. Their chapter samples scholarship on NSSI and communication, asking to what extent researchers have examined possible links between media consumption and self-injury, on one hand, and to what extent communication theories have been used to explain that relationship, on the other.

I close the book with some reflections about ways that we might think differently about NSSI and how we might express those thoughts to patients, to healthcare providers, to students and professional researchers, and to our communities at large. Drawing upon my personal exploration of Buddhist philosophy, I suggest that we reconsider our perceptions of identity, stigma, compassion, and universal suffering in light of social conditions precipitating and conditioning NSSI.

Having provided a brief overview of this book's contents, I return to my student's words:

> I spent years trying to make sure my cuts and scars were always covered, but I don't anymore. I decided that it was nobody's business but my own, and that I shouldn't have to make myself uncomfortable wearing long sleeves or pants when I don't want to just for the sake of making everyone around me comfortable.

These are the words of a confident young woman. She is not exactly the same person who forbade me from using her interview last year. This year, she took her story back, carefully considered each word and phrase, red-lined and rewrote until the text fully represents what she thinks and feels. Somewhere along the way, she became more empowered. By working with her, asking her to reconsider her participation, and giving her full control over the final edit of her words, I participated in a small way in that empowerment.

For me, "empowerment" means the ability to make informed decisions for oneself without fear of retribution. That's what this book is all about. By asking *how* NSSI is communicated about, *what* NSSI is communicating, and how can we do a better job in communicating *about* NSSI, this book's fundamental purpose is to empower individuals who self-injure as well as their families, friends, healthcare providers, and communities in communicating *better* about NSSI. Again, as editor, I challenge you, the reader, to find something useful in each chapter.

Warren Bareiss

WORKS CITED

Anderson, Benedict. *Imagined Communities: Reflections on the Origin and Spread of Nationalism*. London: Verso Books, 1983.

Frank, Arthur W. *The Wounded Storyteller: Body, Illness, and Ethics*. Chicago: University of Chicago Press, 2013. (Original work published in 1995).

International Society for the Study of Self-Injury. "Mission Statement." https://itriples.org/ (accessed April 5, 2020).

Chapter 1

Non-Suicidal Self-Injury

Communicating in Chaos

Marta Carvalhal and Nicole S. Parrish

The International Society for the Study of Self-Injury (ISSS) defines non-suicidal self-injury (NSSI) as "the deliberate, self-inflicted damage of body tissue without suicidal intent and for purposes not socially or culturally sanctioned" (2019).[1] Although NSSI has received much attention over the past twenty years, it is not new. The first clinical case report was published in 1846 describing a 48-year-old, widowed woman who enucleated both of her eyes because she felt guilt-ridden (Khan et al. 1985), and in 1896, Gould and Pyle described cases of young girls who repeatedly inserted needles and other sharp objects into their skin.

NSSI presents itself in many forms in many different types of patients, and the motivation behind these behaviors must be viewed within the context of the psychological, social, medical, and environmental factors pertinent to each patient. Is NSSI a form of communication? If so, what are those who self-injure saying? Are they aware that their behavior carries meaning beyond the immediate behavior? Who are these individuals, and how do we as healthcare professionals communicate with them effectively? In this chapter, we will review these questions and others by examining published literature in light of our experience as healthcare professionals treating NSSI individuals.

Throughout this chapter, we provide examples of NSSI that we have encountered and discuss what we have learned about the link between communication and NSSI. In doing so, we aim to provide a general understanding of NSSI with a primary focus on interpersonal and intrapersonal communication—both intentional and unintentional. Following a discussion of NSSI functions, we will discuss established methods of working with

NSSI patients and describe our approach to fostering mindfulness in patients as a way of redirecting patients' responses away from self-harm and toward self-awareness.

The primary function of people who use NSSI is not always communication. Nevertheless, some primary functions may indirectly communicate the needs of the individuals and the purpose of their behavior. It is important that we understand how people who self-injure function in order to achieve therapeutic rapport.

First, a few definitions are in order. By "intrapersonal communication" we mean a person's internal language that generally serves to enhance self-awareness, self-management, and self-confidence. "Interpersonal communication," on the other hand, is used to denote communication between the patient and others which is essential to a patient's ability to receive help and support, to cooperate with others, and to form healthy relationships (Turner et al. 2012). When we discuss "mindfulness," we mean focusing on the present moment, being aware of one's body, breathing, and emotions.

Patients' motivation for NSSI might not be immediately clear to themselves or their loved ones. It is important that healthcare providers be a source of compassion and knowledge to help patients achieve knowledge and clarification they need to understand their behavior. Healthcare providers must develop a positive therapeutic alliance with NSSI patients and carefully step into their world to learn who they are as people and what the world looks and feels like through their eyes. Patient background, such as developmental and social history, will provide many clues as will other areas of exploration such as medical history, family history, and social history (Townsend and Morgan 2000; van der Kolk et al. 2015).

Social history is a particularly important part of evaluating patients who engage in NSSI behaviors. Social history encompasses a broad range of topics including employment, current housing type, who lives at home, special skills and hobbies, current and past romantic relationships, struggles growing up, current stressors, history of trauma, family history of mental illness, and spirituality.

A female patient of twenty-five years of age, for example, who describes a dozen romantic relationships over the last few years, all beginning fast, all ending fast, and all involving a pattern of intense emotion and conflict can provide a wealth of information about who she is, how she handles interpersonal relationships, stress, and conflict and the effect that these relationships have had on her as she learned to navigate her world as a young adult. These details will help the healthcare provider work with the patient to piece together factors that might be driving the patient to inflict self-harm. Then, the task of helping the patient gain personal insight pertaining to these factors begins. The healthcare provider works to offer a safe environment for the patient to learn to practice more appropriate ways of communicating needs and emotions to herself and others, with the goal of eventually replacing NSSI altogether.

At the intrapersonal level, NSSI is often described by patients and NSSI researchers as a coping mechanism used for temporary relief of emotional distress (Klonsky 2007). NSSI can also be a way to manage emotional or physical pain or to elicit pain (Ebrinc et al. 2008). Some examples of immediate outcomes include feeling pleasure, avoiding or suppressing negative feelings, avoiding or suppressing painful images or memories, escaping from or suppressing a twilight or numb state, punishing oneself, making oneself unattractive, demonstrating strength to oneself or others, and avoiding doing something unpleasant.

At the interpersonal level, individuals can use NSSI as a means of avoiding being with others, as a form of punishment by making others feel guilty (Klonsky 2007), and/or an effort to obtain the necessary attention from others so that they can get the help they need or obtain the social connections they are lacking. Attention seeking, however, is a motive that must be discussed with care. We have often heard well-meaning healthcare providers describe patients who self-injure with a tone of annoyance—"they just want attention"—and label the patient as "manipulative." Humans are social creatures, and the desire to be loved, cared for, and be part of a group is unarguably a human trait. Perhaps it is better to say these patients "need" attention. All humans need to be attended to by others at various points in life, especially during crises. Many patients do, indeed, need for the people around them to look their way and recognize the distress or pain under the surface and then help them without unnecessary skeptical judgment.

PATIENT MOTIVATION AS OPPORTUNITIES FOR RAPPORT BUILDING

Patients, more often than not, have several underlying motivations for NSSI and are broadly practicing both intrapersonal and interpersonal communication with these behaviors (see, for example, Turner et al. 2012). Figure 1.1 illustrates several interrelated functions and communicative aspects of NSSI which we will address in this section within umbrella issues of dissociation, reduction of negative thoughts and emotions, and self-punishment.

Controlling Dissociative Episodes

NSSI sometimes functions to initiate or stop episodes of dissociation. Dissociation is "characterized by a disruption of and/or discontinuity in the

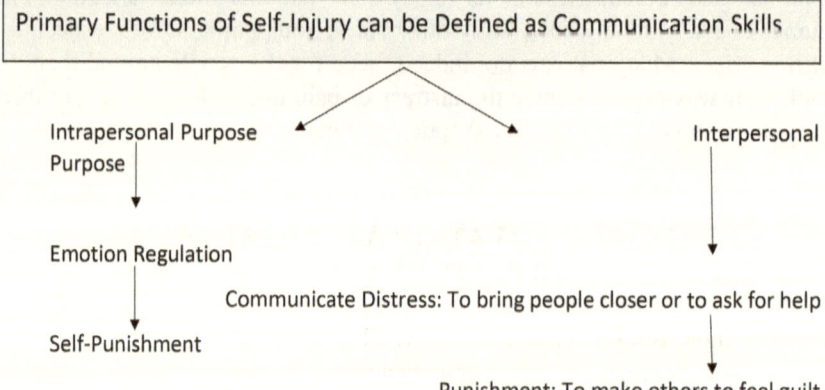

Figure 1.1 Functions of NSSI. *Source*: ©Copyright-Carvalhal.

normal integration of consciousness, memory, identity, emotion, perception, body representation, motor control, and behavior" (American Psychiatric Association 2013, p. 291). In addition, some people report that they feel numb or dead when they dissociate. They also may not be aware of why they're having dissociative episodes. Dissociation often happens to those who have experienced trauma, abuse, and/or other underlying mental illnesses such as depression and anxiety. In contrast to how dissociation feels, self-injury provides a sense of being real, being alive, and of feeling something (Horne and Csipke 2009).

Barbara[2], for example, was a fifteen-year-old patient who used a razor to carve "WaKe UP" on her arm to avoid dissociation. Reading the words "WaKe UP" on Barbara's skin, Marta (coauthor of this chapter) hypothesized that something had happened to numb Barbara's emotions and that Barbara was cutting herself so that she could feel something again. Indeed, as Marta learned, Barbara had been suffering from severe depression and lived in a chaotic household where she was often at the receiving end of criticism and name calling. One day, the chaos of the household erupted into physical violence, and Barbara witnessed the death of a parent. Not yet in therapy, she found it difficult to feel emotions in general, and she understandably felt a general lack of pleasure with life. Cutting, in her case, would stop dissociation as a means of feeling emotionally numb.

In another case, Tina—25-year-old female patient—was treated in our ED. Tina reported that she cut so that she could "feel something . . . anything." She said that a feeling of numbness often overcame her and that she felt like she was not real or not awake. Her dissociative episodes had started in her early teens after being subjected to several years of sexual abuse at the hands of her mother's boyfriend. She was diagnosed with PTSD and had undergone several medication trials of various antidepressants to target her mood symptoms and anxiety. She explained that triggers, such as seeing a man at the playground with a teenage or a child, would make her freeze and go into "a trance for what seems like forever." Later she would return home and cut her legs to get herself back "into the world" so that she could feel awake again and finish her homework. She wore winter style clothing all year to cover her scars and reported that she would rather have scars than feel dead all the time: "It is how I tell myself I am still alive."

Careful building of therapeutic rapport, beginning during initial encounters can help patients like Tina and Barbara to begin the journey to healing. Investigation into the cause of dissociation by empathetic and open communication provides examples of appropriate behavior and communication techniques. The healthcare provider becomes a role model for both interpersonal and intrapersonal communication skill building that can lead to healing and strength in tackling difficulties moving forward in life. We will return to this theme later in this chapter.

Reducing Negative Emotions

Another common function of NSSI is to reduce or relieve stress from pent-up emotions (Hack and Martin 2018). We have worked with several individuals who cut their legs, arms, or other areas concealed under clothing. These patients often shared a sense reduced stress and anxiety after the NSSI behavior. Cutting allowed them to get back to their day and complete tasks such as a school assignment or an objective at work.

Reducing negative emotions appears, on the surface, to be the opposite of controlling dissociative episodes. While Tina was cutting to *feel* emotion, this function is to *decrease* emotions. However, at the core of these two seemingly opposing functions is the fact that these patients need emotional regulation. For some patients, NSSI temporarily relieves intense feelings, stress, pressures, sadness or anxiety, creating a sense of peace. Such emotional distress for NSSI patients can lead to emotional dysregulation (Andover and Morris 2014). Therefore, individuals who struggle with anxiety may use NSSI as a way to control overwhelming distress.

Self-injuring patients can be high-functioning individuals, as was the situation with Janine—a twenty-year old college student who cut her foot with a razor. Janine had been frequently making several superficial small cuts in order to release anxiety and stress she felt in her academic life. This behavior had started in late middle school and was reinforced by the immediate relief she felt after each cut. As life stressors went from childhood problems to more adult problems, the cuts got bigger and a little deeper.

Janine presented to therapy having had years of reinforcement of her behavior, and now, she was unable to stop the urges. She had no other methods to help regulate her emotions in response to stress. Through therapy, Janine developed the understanding—an "ah ha moment"—that NSSI seemed to allow her to refocus herself on her academic studies. The behavior was reinforced by the immediate relaxation she experienced and the overall success she attained academically. Her cutting was a self-soothing technique, as she insightfully realized in session one day. It was as if she had been cutting to tell herself "I'm all right. See, now everything is better. I can now complete my work. I am relaxed now."

The pain analgesia/opiate hypothesis of NSSI has intrigued many researchers over the years and has consistently appeared in cases across nationalities and genders (Groschwitz and Plener 2012), with patients reporting very little or no pain during their act of self-injury. In a sense, this is not very different from how we handle physical pain at times. Imagine, for a moment, that you have just stubbed your toe on your bedroom dresser. In reaction to this, you bite your lip and clench your fists in an attempt to divert attention away from the throbbing pain of your mangled toe. Having had some success with this technique, you are likely to remind yourself that it works to deflect attention from the greater pain on further occasions until it becomes second nature.

Likewise, cutting the skin can serve to redirect attention away from the intense emotional pain located within oneself; however, unlike the toe pain that will quickly subside and generally go away completely, once the pain from the razor cuts fades into memory, the masked emotional pain continues and comes back to the surface. It is our job as healthcare providers to help patients understand the function NSSI serves for them and to redirect responses to stress, trauma, and so forth by teaching appropriate coping skills to replace NSSI via appropriate intrapersonal reminders.

Guided imagery scripts are frequently employed in therapy sessions to teach regulation of emotionally distressing experiences. A consistent decrease in physiological arousal occurs when patients work through an NSSI imagery script, similar to what occurs when a patient performs NSSI to decrease anxiety or distress (Welch 2008). Patients struggling with emotion dysregulation receive a great benefit from the practice of guided imagery or self-guided imagery.

Marta taught Janine mindfulness and emotion regulation skills, beginning with focus on her breathing. Once relaxed, Janine was guided through an imaginary scene, such as a forest, as she focused on deep breathing (Creswell et al. 2016), consequently, relaxing her body. The scenery was described in great detail to help Janine stay focused and also engage all of Janine's senses. Janine would eventually learn to replace cutting with guided imagery where she would go back to the forest in her mind as she calmed her emotions and relaxed her body.

Reducing Negative Thoughts

Just as our patients use NSSI to divert attention away from emotional pain or anxiety, NSSI also can function as a way to seek relief from negative thoughts. Intrapersonal communication, again, is used by the patient harboring a negative self-perception. For example, David was a patient in his twenties who had suffered extensive sexual abuse from a relative from the age of six until his early teens. When he first arrived for treatment, David had never told anyone about the abuse. Old scars were visible all over David's upper arms. On his left arm, David had a scar that spelled out "HATE." On his right arm, he had extensive parallel cuttings.

The drive behind this particular NSSI was eventually identified by David as a means to stop the thoughts of shame, betrayal, and intrusive memories of the abuse. David came to realize that he was communicating self-hatred *intra*personally and at the same time was asking for help *inter*personally. David carved words into his skin because he was unable to verbalize "I hate him" or "I hate myself."

A family meeting was facilitated with David and his mother. When David told his mother what had happened, she did not show any compassion or understanding. She also needed help in communicating and expressing her emotions and thoughts in a constructive way. Most likely, she was emotionally disconnected due to a history of abuse, too. Upon discharge, David was motivated to continue outpatient therapy. His mother, however, did not see the need for family therapy.

As mentioned previously, patients' motivation for performing NSSI might not be immediately clear to themselves. Indeed, many teenagers feel that their acts of NSSI are not "serious" and or that they are managing the issues just fine on their own (Fortune et al. 2008). Although we as healthcare providers can readily interpret the word "HATE" carved on a young person's arm as an unconscious form of communication, the patient might not recognize this until the start of therapy.

Self-Punishment

Some self-injurers punish themselves for having strong feelings of self-hatred which they were usually not allowed to express to others as children or young adults. Others use NSSI because they perceive themselves as unlovable (Hack and Martin 2018).

While David self-injured to reduce negative thoughts, he also was likely cutting as a means of self-punishment—hence, the double meaning of the word "HATE." David felt hate toward his family member for sexually abusing him—hate which he was unable to express and felt uncomfortable feeling, so he projected the hate back onto himself. He often had blamed himself and was ashamed of himself. This was a difficult concept for David. Why would he punish himself and hate himself when the person who had sexually abused him should have received the hate and punishment?

Many patients who we have treated experience this complex situation wherein the patient hates a close relative who was supposed to be protective, and yet, the patient is also uncomfortable in feeling that hate. Such cognitive dissonance leads to confusion about where to target blame. For example, a child that lives in a home with an abusive, alcoholic mother will experience periods of intense emotions toward the parent. Sometimes, that emotion is hatred toward the parent. Other times, the emotion is love because the parent provides a birthday present, a hug, or a favorite meal as well needed validation.

In the child's mind, it is unacceptable to hate the parent for two reasons. First, the child has learned that expressing aggression or negative emotions toward the alcoholic parent often leads to physical violence and even physical punishment of the child, and this certainly is to be avoided. Second, the child has been taught that they should love the parent, and it doesn't feel "right" to both love and hate a person. Therefore, hatred must be dealt with in another way. The child takes the hate and projects it back on themselves through punishment, much like David likely did in our earlier example. Sometimes that punishment eventually takes the form of NSSI in the present or later in life.

In some cases, this self-hatred stems from a distortion of self: "Bad people deserve to be punished, and I am a bad person," is often an underlying core belief of these patients and a theme that we hear quite often. The self-punishment hypothesis of NSSI has been most strongly linked to repeated abuse and criticism by others (Fortune et al. 2016).

We have observed and treated several patients over the years who have carved various words into their skin, for example, "bad," "faggot," and—as we have discussed above—"hate." These words not only express how patients felt about themselves, but also how they perceived the way that the world views them.

It is important to notice that self-punishment through NSSI can take other forms, however. For example, few years ago while in the intensive medical management unit of a psychiatric ward, Jim—an elderly patient with schizoaffective disorder—stated that he needed to cut off his genitalia because an angel had told him to do so. He demanded to be released from the hospital so that he could follow through with the will of God. Later, as he wept in his room, he insisted that he was being held against his will and that he would be damned for eternity for not following through with his holy instructions. Jim later revealed that he felt he had sinned in many ways during his life, and his depression appeared to stem from his guilt regarding those prior sins. Jim's desire to cut off his genitalia was his means of redemption. His psychotic state certainly influenced his ideas and clouded his judgment and insight, and his urge to perform NSSI behavior was intense and difficult to treat, not unlike the other patients mentioned in this section.

Such cases of urges influenced by psychosis can be particularly devastating and can even lead to accidental death. After treatment with antipsychotic therapy was initiated, Jim was able to participate in therapy regarding his depressive symptoms. Sadly, this elderly gentleman had many episodes of relapse into psychotic states over the course of his life due to medication nonadherence as is typical with schizophrenia spectrum disorders, and even after treatment with antipsychotics, he would return to our inpatient unit with the urge to perform the same NSSI behavior again and again.

As the preceding cases illustrate, healthcare providers must attempt to understand how people with NSSI function, how they view themselves. and how they view and engage with the world in order to achieve successful therapeutic communication. Trust is essential if the patient is to feel safe in communicating directly through words, rather than indirectly via NSSI. Information provided by the patient should be received in a nonjudgmental fashion and with the utmost care given to patient confidentiality.

NEUROSCIENCE AND NSSI

Many patients presented thus far have a history of trauma, such as Barbara, who endured years of emotional abuse, and Tina and David, who experienced sexual abuse. Greeson (2008) found that behaviors of individuals like Barbara, Tina, and David are often strongly influenced by the sympathetic nervous system (SNS) which increases emotional arousal. The SNS is more commonly referred to the "fight or flight" system; however, we will refer to it as the *emotional mind*—a common term used in dialectic behavioral therapy (DBT) (see Linehan 1993a).

The *emotional mind* is an intense and impulsive emotional state that patients can become enveloped in when under stress. It is reactive and unregulated. Needing to fight or flee immediately, it acts impulsively to achieve immediate resolution. In contrast, the *rational mind* is the parasympathetic nervous system (PNS). The PNS is the center for insight and judgment, the capacity of making decision. It also is the memorization and learning area of the brain. The third mind—the *wise mind*—is awareness of the present moment. The *wise mind* balances between the *emotional mind* and *the rational mind* (Linehan 1993a).

When Janine—the college student mentioned previously—first started cutting, she experienced immediate distress relief. Intense emotion activated the SNS. Janine felt tense as her muscles stiffened and her heart beat faster in response to stress. The impulse to relieve the stress led Janine to make shallow cuts and then to cut more deeply. Janine eventually revealed through therapy that she noticed that seemingly insignificant stressors to others eventually resulted in her cutting herself. It seemed that her SNS was overactive; her emotional mind was in control so that the delicate balance of her nervous system had become disrupted over time. In individuals who have experienced multiple traumas, the balance of the nervous system can tilt immediately, or soon afterward, toward SNS domination. This is thought to produce a neurochemical imbalance in the brain primarily of serotonin. Research demonstrates that individuals who self-mutilate have decreased serotonin levels, and it is thought that low serotonin levels go on to increase the risk of self-harm and anger (Groschwitz and Plener 2012).

As individuals develop new coping skills such as mindfulness, meditation, and relaxation, they start using the PNS more often (Greeson 2008). This might be because therapy intervention helps the individual put their nervous system back into a state of balance. It is possible that through therapy—just like with medications such as antidepressants—serotonin levels increase. The *emotional mind* and the *wise mind* can thus be thought of in biological terms.

On one hand, understanding the biology and neurochemistry helps us in the mental health professions to comprehend the power of reinforcement

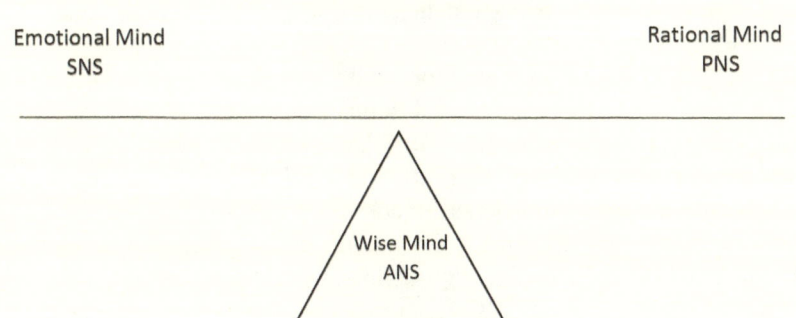

Figure 1.2 *Source*: ©Copyright-Carvalhal.

produced by NSSI. On the other hand, assessment of the functions of NSSI and the patient's communication skills allows us to effectively help patients work toward centering themselves—bringing balance into their lives and hopefully, back into their brain's chemistry (Figure 1.2).

TEACHING COMMUNICATION SKILLS VIA DIALECTICAL BEHAVIORAL THERAPY

Sadly, the actions of patients who self-injure can result in unintended responses from people, and the support system that patients attempt to draw upon may dissipate as a result. As discussed earlier, it is not uncommon to hear patients who self-injure labeled as "attention seekers," even by healthcare providers. This label suggests that acts of NSSI are not serious and might imply that the patient does not require clinical attention and treatment. For example, while Jim's desire to cut off his genitalia is more easily seen as needing direct clinical intervention, Janine's cuts did not reach the attention of a therapist until her cuts were very deep and no longer able to be covered. The clinician must be cautious to avoid communicating such negative labels or further supporting some patients' perception that their behavior is not very serious.

DBT has strong support as an important strategy for treating NSSI (Andover and Morris 2014). This form of therapy is divided in four modules: *Core mindfulness* is the foundation of the other modules; if the individual is not mindful, she or he will not be able to utilize the other skills. *Emotion regulation skills* teach the individual to be aware of their emotions and manage it in a productive way. *Interpersonal skills* teach how to communicate needs and wants in an effective way without compromising self-values. *Distress tolerance skills* teach how to survive crisis situations without making them worse. Most NSSI patients have deficits in one or more of these areas.

As a form of cognitive behavioral therapy, DBT teaches patients new skills and strategies to handle their emotions and stress (Linehan 1993b). The goal for patients, such as those mentioned in this chapter, is to eventually replace acts of NSSI with these new skills—to achieve a balance where the *wise mind* is not being pushed aside by the *emotional mind* any longer. Some common skills that we use with our patients include mindfulness, emotional regulation, distress tolerance, and interpersonal communication strategies. Treatment can take place in both individual and group therapy settings.

An example of our use of DBT was when a patient, JoAnne, developed dissociative identity disorder after suffering multiple types of abuse and trauma growing up, much like Barbara and Tina had experienced. The use of two key concepts of DBT—*radical acceptance* and *mindfulness*—were particularly helpful during therapy with this patient. *Radical acceptance* is letting go of fighting reality (Linehan 1993b). "Radical" means that the acceptance has to come from deep within and has to be complete. "Acceptance" is the preferred path out of one's personal hell. It is the way to turn suffering that cannot be tolerated into pain that can be tolerated. Pain is part of living; it can be emotional, and it can be physical. As Linehan (ibid.) explains, "Acceptance is acknowledging what is. To accept something is not the same as judging that it is good or approving of it. Acceptance is turning my suffering into pain that I can endure" (p. 102). Generally, in treating patients like JoAnne, Marta explains to the patient that radical acceptance is the first step toward their freedom.

Working with JoAnne in the ED, Marta asked JoAnne to visualize herself standing in a pool of mud trying to move forward, but not being able to due to the fact that she has not accepted the unpleasant and painful things that happened in the past. Next, Marta reinforced that acceptance is just acknowledging that these events happened; it does not mean that it was fair or we are judging it as good or bad.

From that point, JoAnne was introduced to the concept of being mindful. *Mindfulness* means intentionally living with awareness in the present, without judging or rejecting the moment and without attachment to the moment (Linehan 1993b). Deep breathing and mindfulness skills stimulate the vagus nerve which, in turn, helps the body to relax by activating the PNS (Creswell et al. 2016). In her treatment of JoAnne, Marta explained that that in order to move forward and get out of the thick mud, JoAnne would have to practice radical acceptance and mindfulness skills.

Amid the confusion and sounds of the ED, Marta provided guided relaxation and deep breathing so that JoAnne was able to calm her nervous system, regulate her emotions, and channel her energy toward talking with Marta about her feelings and needs. From the ED, JoAnne was transferred to an inpatient facility where she received dialectical behavioral therapy in combination with pharmacological treatment.

COMMUNICATING WITH NSSI PATIENTS

When engaging with patients who self-injure, we try to redirect them from dominance of SNS toward skills that will enhance the PNS.

Due to the many possible causes of NSSI, we deal with a complex assortment of sub-populations, yet we tend to approach each case with the same general questions: Are they struggling to accept the situation that they are in and to communicate their fear, anger, insecurity in a more beneficial and productive way? Are they aware of the issues—intrapersonal or interpersonal—they are communicating through NSSI?

We attempt to answer those general issues by trying to ascertain details specific to each case. Consequently, we ask specific questions related to each patient: What was the purpose for your cutting or burning? How did it help you improve the moment? How did you feel before *punching*? How did you feel after *scratching*? What were you trying to *communicate*? The purpose of these questions as stated above, is to foster mindfulness in patients as a way of redirecting their responses away from self-harm toward self-awareness and of helping patients make connections with the functions of NSSI, their emotions, and their behavior.

Once, for example, Armond—a visiting international college student—was burning himself with lit cigarettes. Marta asked questions about motivations and functions of Armond's behavior. This opened the door for dialog. Afterward, Armond felt comfortable in sharing the struggle of new culture, family pressure, and fear of failure.

Another example was Terry, a patient who cut "faggot" in his arm. Marta started the conversation with him by asking, "Do you believe you are a faggot or do you believe it when people call you a faggot?" Next, she asked Terry how NSSI helped him to improve the situation by using the series of questions mentioned in the above paragraph. After this initial contact with Armond, Terry, and any other patient, we start teaching DBT to optimize treatment and decrease recidivism.

CONCLUDING THOUGHTS

We started this chapter with some questions: Is NSSI a form of communication? If so, what are these individuals trying to say? How do we as healthcare professionals communicate with patients who self-injure effectively? As we discussed throughout this chapter, in our experience, among the most important reasons to practice NSSI is the need for intrapersonal or interpersonal communication. Most of the individuals we have worked with are not aware of the communication motivation behind their NSSI behaviors. Sometimes, even their healthcare professionals are not aware of its communication purposes.

Healthcare professionals and researchers have come a long way since Favazza (1996) first published, *Bodies Under Siege*. We must inform and teach these new findings to individuals who use NSSI and to those who care for them.

Lastly, we have learned over the years to practice mindfulness ourselves, for example, engaging in deep breathing skills daily. We embrace DBT modules in our personal and professional lives. At the professional level, we are prone to our own forms of harmful behaviors such as overworking, not taking of ourselves, always putting others always of us, and so on. Hopefully, this chapter not only helps healthcare providers treat their patients, but also, makes them aware of the need to live mindfully themselves.

NOTES

1. Abbreviations specific to this chapter: DBT (dialectic behavioral therapy), SNS (sympathetic nervous system), PNS (the parasympathetic nervous system).
2. All patient names in this chapter are pseudonyms.

WORKS CITED

American Psychiatric Association. *Diagnostic and Statistical Manual of Mental Disorders* (5th ed.). Arlington, VA: American Psychiatric Publishing, 2013.

Andover, Margaret, S. Blair, and W. Morris. "Expanding and Clarifying the Role of Emotion Regulation in Nonsuicidal Self-Injury." *Canadian Journal of Psychiatry* 59, no. 11 (2014): 569–575.

Creswell, J. David, Adrienne A. Taren, Emily K. Lindsay, Carol M. Greco, Peter J. Gianaros, April Fairgrieve, Anna L. Marsland, Kirk Warren Brown, Baldwin M. Way, Rhonda K. Rosen, and Jennifer L. Ferris. "Alterations in Resting-State Functional Connectivity Link Mindfulness Meditation with Reduced Interleukin-6: A Randomized Controlled Trial." *Biological Psychiatry* 80, no. 1 (2016): 53–61.

Ebrinc, Servet, Umit B. Semiz, Cengiz Basoglu, Mesut Cetin, Mehmet Y. Agargun, Ayhan Algul, and Alpay Ates. "Self-Mutilating Behavior in Patients with Dissociative Disorders: The Role of Innate Hypnotic Capacity." *Israel Journal of Psychiatry and Related Sciences* 45, no. 1 (2008): 39–48.

Favazza, Armondo. *Bodies Under Siege: Self-Mutilation and Body Modification in Culture and Psychiatry* (2nd ed.). Baltimore: The John Hopkins University Press, 1996.

Fortune, Sarah, David Cottrell, and Sarah Fife. "Family Factors Associated with Adolescent Self-Harm: A Narrative Review." *Journal of Family Therapy* 32, no. 2 (2016): 226–256.

Fortune, Sarah, Julia Sinclair, and Keith Hawton. "Help-Seeking Before and After Episodes of Self-Harm: A Descriptive Study in School Pupils in England." *BMC Public Health* 8, no. 1 (2008): 369.

Gould, George M., and Walter L. Pyle. *Anomalies and Curiosities of Medicine*. Sydney: Wentworth Press, Reprint (1896) 2016.

Greeson, Jeffrey M. "Mindfulness Research Update: 2008." *Journal of Evidence-Based Integrative Medicine* 14, no. 1 (2008): 10–18.

Groschwitz, Rebecca C., and Paul L. Plener. "The Neurobiology of Non-Suicidal Self-Injury (NSSI): A Review." *Suicidology Online* 3 (2012): 24–32.

Hack, Jessica, and Graham Martin. "Expressed Emotion, Shame, and Non-Suicidal Self-Injury." *International Journal of Environmental Research and Public Health* 15, no. 5 (2018): 890.

Horne, Outi, and Emise Csipke. "From Feeling Too Little and Too Much, to Feeling More and Less? A Nonparadoxical Theory of the Functions of Self-Harm." *Qualitative Health Research* 19, no. 5 (2009): 655–667.

International Society for the Study of Self-Mutilation. "What Is Nonsuicidal Self-Injury?" https://itriples.org/about-self-injury/what-is-self-injury/

Khan, Jemshed A., Lucinda Buescher, Carl H. Ide, and Ben Pettigrove. "Medical Management of Self-Enucleation." *Archives of Ophthalmology* 103, no. 3 (1985): 386–389.

Klonsky, E. David. "The Functions of Deliberate Self-Injury: A Review of the Evidence." *Clinical Psychology Review* 27, no. 2 (2007): 226–239.

Linehan, Marsha M. *Skills Training Manual for Treating Borderline Personality Disorder*. New York: The Guilford Press, 1993a.

Linehan, Marsha M. *Cognitive-Behavioral Treatment of Borderline Personality Disorder*. New York: The Guilford Press, 1993b.

Townsend, Mary E., and Karyn I. Morgan. *Psychiatric Mental Health Nursing: Concepts of Care in Evidence-Based Practice*. Philadelphia: F.A Davis. Co., 2000.

Turner, Brianna J., Alexander L. Chapman, and Brianne K. Layden. "Intrapersonal and Interpersonal Functions of Nonsuicidal Self-Injury: Associations with Emotional and Social Functioning." *Suicide Life Threat Behavior* 42, no. 1 (2012): 36–55.

van der Kolk, Bessel. *The Body Keeps the Score: Brain, Mind, and Body in the Healing of Trauma*. London: Penguin Books, 2015.

Welch, Stacy Shaw, Marsha M. Linehan, Patrick Sylvers, Jesse Chittams, and Shireen L. Rizvi. "Emotional Responses to Self-Injury Imagery Among Adults with Borderline Personality Disorder." *Journal of Counseling and Clinical Psychology* 76, no. 1 (2008): 45–51.

Chapter 2

Self-Regulatory Communication in the Treatment of Self-Injury

Development and Maintenance of Therapeutic Rapport

John L. Levitt

INTRODUCTION

Non-suicidal self-injury (NSSI) represents considerable challenges for healthcare professionals (Klonsky 2009; Nock 2010).[1] NSSI behaviors themselves—for example, cutting, burning, and banging—are counterintuitive for most people, including professionals. The notion that one should intentionally cause bodily injury to feel better, cope, communicate to others, and so forth, is not one that most individuals tend to embrace.

NSSI represents complex, multi-determined symptom constellations that are often accompanied by a number of psychological problems including eating disorders (e.g., Levitt 2005; Levitt and Sansone 2002; Levitt et al. 2004; Sansone and Levitt 2002), personality disorders, major depression, anxiety disorders, substance abuse, posttraumatic stress disorder, schizophrenia (see Haw et al. 2001; Herpertz et al. 1997; Klonsky et al. 2003; Klonsky 2009; Klonsky and Muehlenkamp 2007; Zlotnick et al. 1999), and sexual abuse (Vanderlinden and Vandereycken 1997). Though NSSI symptoms are frequently found in adolescent and adult women, research indicates an increased prevalence of such symptoms in older women and in males of various ages (Nock 2010).

Nock (2010) suggests that 13 percent to 45 percent of adolescents and 4 percent of adults report having deliberately self-harmed during their lifetime (344) (see also, Klonsky 2007, 2009; Lloyd-Richardson et al. 2007), and other studies indicate that the general prevalence of self-injury among outpatient clients or inpatient clients can be as high as 25 percent (Levitt and Sansone 2002; Sansone and Levitt 2002; Levitt et al. 2004). Some authors have suggested that the percentage of individuals who cut themselves might be similar to those who have anorexia nervosa (Conterio and Lader 1998; Levenkron 1998). In addition, the self-injury literature indicates that the NSSI rate may be as high as 35 percent to 40 percent in the eating disorder population (Favazza 1987, p. 204). Similar findings are emerging in the area of substance abuse (Moran et al. 2015).

Some difficulties in identifying the prevalence of self-harming behaviors in clients presenting with other issues is due to the private, secretive nature of NSSI, the often accompanying shame in the client who self-harms for merely having the problem, and the lack of easy-to-use assessment tools suitable for examining both self-injury and other behaviors in a clinical setting (see, for example, Sansone and Sansone 2002). Indeed, there are few tools and interventional approaches designed to address the multi-symptomatic client who presents with NSSI.

Similarly, there are few treatment approaches specifically designed to simultaneously address both NSSI behaviors and another specific disorder. While most authors emphasize that treatment approaches should be tailored and sequentially implemented on an individual basis (Andersen 1985; Garner and Needleman 1997), the literature is relatively unclear as to how one might undertake this among NSSI clients presenting with a possibly more than one symptom cluster (Levitt and Sansone 2002; Levitt et al. 2004; Wonderlich et al. 2002).

A rare exception in the literature, Vanderlinden and Vandereycken (1997) describe self-harming behaviors as sequelae of traumatic life events in the histories of clients with eating disorders. These authors present an excellent overview of trauma and impulse dyscontrol, which subsequently lead to self-injury, and they make specific suggestions regarding the management of self-injurious behaviors (87–89). This is especially important as research increasingly suggests that a significant number of individuals seeking services in the healthcare system report histories of trauma and abuse. Consequently, it is likely that these challenging clients will seek and require services, and professionals will need to develop effective rapport with them in ways that will enhance outcomes.

This chapter is designed to briefly explore the general functions of NSSI and their impact on the development of therapeutic rapport and communication. It is not intended to replace more thorough discussions of these functions (e.g., Klonsky 2009; Klonsky and Muehlenkamp 2007; Nock 2010), but to illustrate their impact on communication between therapist and client as they develop and potentially impact the working relationship. Ideas relevant to how the NSSI behaviors function within the relationship and various options for addressing them are also presented.

In the following sections of this chapter, the functions of NSSI will be briefly reviewed followed by a description of the Self-Regulatory Approach (SRA) as it pertains to NSSI. Particular focus will be on the impact of the various elements of the SRA as they potentially impact the therapeutic relationship. Following that, the stages and elements involved with developing a therapeutic relationship are briefly described. Short descriptions of potential scenarios that might be experienced in treatment are presented.[2]

FUNCTIONS OF NSSI BEHAVIORS

To best understand NSSI's impact on the therapeutic arena during relational development, it is useful to understand the general functions that NSSI might provide for clients as they participate in therapeutic communications. Klonsky and associates (Klonsky 2007, 2009; Klonsky and Muehlenkamp 2007) identified seven general functions of NSSI from the literature. Later, they reduced these to three functions, that is, experiential expectations, of NSSI behaviors often exhibited by clients of NSSI of particular clinical import: the first general function, or expectational result, for the client who self-injures is to obtain relief from a negative feelings or a cognitive state; NSSI behaviors are, therefore, performed when an individual is challenged by a need to reduce a negative emotional state or arousal perceived to be *intolerable*. Second, NSSI behaviors are conducted when an individual is confronted with an interpersonal difficulty that is perceived as *unmanageable* or which has activated arousal to the point of perceived unmanageability, regardless of whether it is realistically manageable or not. Third, NSSI behaviors may be performed in order to induce a positive feeling state that is more *desirable*, such as when the behaviors activate endorphins and result in the individual experiencing a sense of euphoria, relief, calm, and so forth. These functions are all dependent upon the uniquely personal view of the client and might not reflect the client's true skill or ability to manage the situations at hand.

The functions described above tend to represent "strategies" in that they are used fairly consistently in similar situations for either interpersonal or intrapersonal benefits. Clearly, however, many clients present with NSSI behaviors that serve more than one function. In fact, in a recent meta-analysis (Taylor et al. 2018), intrapersonal functions—especially those concerning emotion regulation—were most commonly reported among these clients. Interpersonal functions (e.g., expressing distress) were less common. This suggests that for many, if not most, clients who engage in NSSI behaviors, those behaviors represent efforts to either regulate difficult emotional experiences or represent an effort to increase emotional experience (such as in the case of depersonalization). For example, an individual who depersonalizes might report instances where he/she feels "numb." NSSI might, in this case, be employed as a means to increase emotional/physical experience or awareness of their bodily self (i.e., pain). The authors suggest that this supports recent focus on the affect regulation models (ibid., 765).

It is important to note, however, that affect is often driven from interpersonal experiences and challenges. For example, interpersonal experiences can generate negative emotional experience or result in the absence of experience such as the case when severe abuse/trauma occurs as described above.

How do the three functions pertaining to factors that are *intolerable*, *unmanageable*, and/or *desirable* impact the transactions between the therapist and client when developing therapeutic rapport, that is, effective communication? The following sections describe the role of NSSI, consistent with the information presented above, as a form of self-regulation and to describe how these self-regulatory behaviors can be used as a form of communication in the therapeutic relational milieu.

NSSI and the SRA

Different perspectives of self-regulation have been discussed in the literature including self-regulated learning, self-control, and self-management (Boekaaerts et al. 2000; Carver and Scheier 1998; Linehan 2003). While some researchers look at self-regulation from the perspective of self-control (Baumeister et al. 1994), others view self-regulation in the context of emotion or affect. Siegel (1999), for example, views emotion as playing a central role in self-regulation, whereas Yates (1991) focuses on self-regulation of affect as central to self-management. Others recognize the impacts of therapy on self-regulation (Endler and Kocovski 2000).

Self-regulation, indeed, represents a concept central to a range of views of understanding the development, maintenance, and change in clients' problems. Self-regulation, however, has several central concepts common among these perceptions (Boekaaerts et al. 2000). Based on this, an approach to understanding, engaging, and treating clients who engage in NSSI—among other symptom presentations—was developed and evaluated: the SRA (Levitt 2005; Levitt and Sansone 2004). The following represents a brief overview of the SRA.

From the SRA perspective, all individuals are intimately involved with managing their internal (i.e., emotional/cognitive) responses in the context of interacting with their environmental demands (i.e., relational transactions). The SRA is intended to offer a framework for delivering treatment to this often comorbid population (i.e., clients presenting with NSSI often also present with comorbid conditions). It is not, however, intended to direct interventions, but rather to function as an organizing approach for clinicians who utilize a variety of clinical and theoretical perspectives. Because comorbidity is very common, the SRA was designed to provide a treatment framework for complex behaviors associated with NSSI (Levitt 2000a, 2000b, 2005).

From the SRA perspective, self-regulation essentially refers to one's ability to maintain a steady or constant behavioral, affective, or psychological state despite ongoing environmental demands. NSSI behaviors tend to create for the client the subjective experience of psychological steadiness (e.g., safety, self-efficacy, and well-being). These behaviors, elected by the client, can be characterized by the degree to which they are repeated and relied upon and the extent to which they are utilized over time. Indeed, in severe cases, NSSI behaviors often exhibit a general "resistance to extinction" (Conterio and Lader 1998; Hsu 1990). That is, the tendency to use NSSI behaviors, even when they have not been employed for extended lengths of time, is often present and elicited by various environmental/relational situations.

From the SRA perspective, NSSI symptoms may serve to protect the individual. In many cases, they may help to manage strong affects, enable the client to tolerate the emotional experience(s), calm or soothe oneself, and/or prevent oneself from being overcome by strong affects such as guilt and shame. It is important to keep in mind that self-regulatory functions serve as a backdrop for other important processes necessary for effective functioning. These can include the development of strategies for obtaining self-approval (i.e., being able to know when something is accomplished and the ability to derive satisfaction from it), understanding connections (i.e., between events, behaviors, and outcomes), experiencing a sense of control, and establishing an internal reward system (see, e.g., Baumeister et al. 1994; Boekaaerts et al. 2000).

Overall, self-regulation enables one to organize the flow of information, giving it meaning and relevance. Self-regulation also helps to develop a belief system about oneself in relation to others, the awareness and skill in predicting the effects one's behavior has on the environment, the skill to manage psychological space (i.e., boundaries), a sense of interpersonal safety, a relationship to one's physical body, and the skill to maintain activities of daily living (Levitt et al. 2004). Given the discussion above regarding functions of self-injury, it is clear that NSSI behavioral strategies can be generated to provide a sense of reliable control or constancy over time and situations and, through constant application, serve to regulate the client.

SELF-REGULATION AND THE STRUCTURAL-PROCESS MODEL

As described above, the SRA represents a way of generally understanding various NSSI behaviors as efforts to self-regulate. The SRA was formulated into a model for organizing the therapeutic relationship, monitoring changes within the therapy milieu, and for developing intervention strategies: the Structural-Process Model (SPM) (Levitt 2003, 2004, 2005; Levitt et al. 2004; Sansone et al. 2004). The elements of the SRA were organized into relatively simple, identifiable areas suitable for both the therapist and

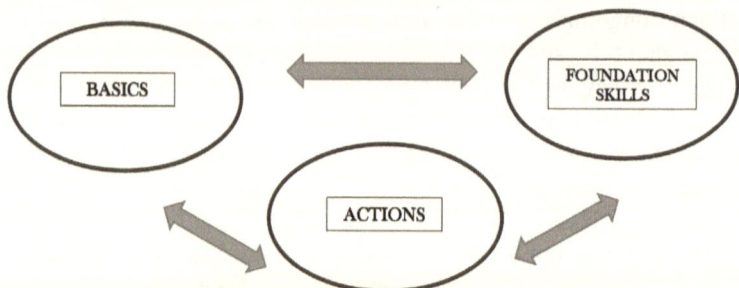

Figure 2.1 **Structural-Process Model.** *Source*: Author created. Levitt, J.L. (2005). "A therapeutic approach to treating the eating disorder/borderline personality disorder patient." *Eating Disorders: The Journal of Treatment and Prevention* vol. 13, no. 1, pp. 109–121.

the client to learn, observe, and effectively apply to change elements of self-regulation as they pertain to problems of living. The model was then clinically evaluated in hospital/outpatient setting to ascertain general efficacy (e.g., Levitt and Sansone 2003; Levitt 2005, 2015). The following represents the elements of the SPM.

A broad responsibility of the therapist is to teach beneficial self-regulation that the client can use in their recovery. We have found that for most clients presenting with NSSI behaviors, the SPM of self-regulation has been proven quite useful. For the therapist, the SPM provides an interpersonal communicative framework and guide for introducing therapeutic content as well as focusing, timing, and pacing interventions (Levitt et al. 2004). For the client, the SPM provides an intrapersonal communicative approach for learning about oneself, identifying areas of difficulty, and for focusing attention during recovery (i.e., reframing one's self-concept as a "student of oneself" rather than a "sick" individual). In this way, the client can view therapy as a student participating in a learning process. Again, in self-regulation, it is important for the client to enter into treatment as an empowered, versus defective, individual (Textbox 2.1).

TEXTBOX 2.1 AN OVERVIEW OF THE STRUCTURAL-PROCESS MODEL SKILL AREAS. ADAPTED BASED ON LEVITT, 2004A

Basics

Safety: is represented by an internal and cognitive awareness of the elements involved in protecting oneself from psychological or behavioral self-injury, risk, or loss.

Security: is exhibited in the skills necessary to identify, avoid, and/or manage high-risk, potentially harmful external relationships or situations.

Physical Well-Being: is reflected in skills demonstrating the ability to recognize and implement self-care behaviors for one's daily physiological and living needs.

Foundation Skills

Communication: reflects the skills involved with self-awareness of "personal" cognitive, emotional, and behavioral information.

Cooperation: is exhibited by the ability to employ self-awareness of personal information and engage it to accomplish goals consistently.

Connectedness: represents the observable ability to remain connected to the therapist and the therapeutic goals exhibited in verbal, behavioral, and interactional behaviors.

Collaboration: is represented by the ability to utilize all of the above Foundation Skills with the therapist and significant others for the purpose of achieving goals important to the client and recovery.

Honesty: is demonstrated by behaviors that reflect the capacity to remain open, able and willing, to disclose both overt and covert information that is relevant and essential for recovery and goal achievement.

Actions

Focus: is reflected in the skills to identify and "target" therapeutic objectives.

Determination: the ability to employ motivation, energy, and personal resources to remain aware of and stay on-task to achieve therapeutic objectives.

Direction: the ability to stay on task over time, settings, situations, and relations, to achieve targeted goals despite obstacles or other interruptions.

Commitment: the ability to maintain a psychological and emotional desire and obligation to the above Action elements.

The SPM consists of three general elements that are used by both the client and therapist for organizing the treatment and monitoring the client's self-regulation: *basics*, *foundation skills*, and *actions*. *Basics* refers to stability and self-care. For example, when initially approaching the client who engages in NSSI, the therapist likely wants to focus on fundamentals including safety, security, and physical well-being. Clients are initially taught and encouraged to explore the *basics* in terms of their own situation, with the therapist's guidance and support. They are encouraged to develop and apply relatively safe thoughts and behaviors toward themselves, and to participate in secure (i.e., not dangerous, threatening, or symptom provoking) interactions with other people and situations.

Additionally, the general goal is for clients to eventually demonstrate appropriate self-care behaviors (e.g., nutrition, sleep, hygiene, exercise, socialization, rest and relaxation, adherence to medical regimens, avoidance of destructive drugs, etc.). For clients who engage in NSSI, this is often a logical, but difficult, first phase of therapy. Indeed, while the therapist needs to be mindful not to push too hard for no self-harming, presenting the *basics* as a way of learning to care for oneself is realistic, appropriate, and understandable for most clients—especially when communicated in such a way that is nonjudgmental and that changes are under the client's control.

Foundation skills generally refer to the ability to monitor and utilize personal information. Thoughts, feelings, and relationship interactions are usually the predominant foci. Elements include skills for communicating with oneself and others to successfully attain goals, utilizing one's own information effectively via intrapersonal communication, remaining involved in treatment, working with others toward being successful, and being consistently honest with oneself and relevant others.

Foundation skills translate the *basics* into therapeutic action. For example, in many cases, the client struggles with modulating their affect arousal without resorting to NSSI behaviors(s). The clinician would tend to ensure that the client had developed some skills to be aware of, identify, and modulate emotional experiences (i.e., personal information) prior to working on more emotionally laden material (e.g., traumatic experience[s]).

Actions refers to those skills and processes that assist the client in being able to stay on-task over time with purpose and conviction. Motivational elements in these clients are identified as skill areas—the ability to sustain attention (focus), for the purpose of obtaining a goal of import to the client (direction) with sustained purpose (determination), and with conviction and resolve (commitment). Action areas provide a means to monitor motivation and on-task behaviors and to reflect elements that suggest to the therapist and client that the client's motivation is on course. The ability to stay on-task is essential for goal attainment. Indeed, while the ebb and flow of NSSI behaviors in recovery are common hallmarks of NSSI, it is important that this be addressed in the recovery process (e.g., Miller 1994; Vanderlinden and Vandereycken 1997). Action skills provide an effective means for monitoring and developing the necessary behaviors and processes I this area necessary for recovery.

SELF-REGULATION AND THE FUNCTION OF "POSITION"

An important aspect of the SPM is the awareness of multidirectional communication between therapist and client. It is vital that the client takes an active role and is an equal participant in treatment (e.g., is self-regulating). In fact, clients who experience therapy as efficacious and successful are somewhat less likely to turn to NSSI (Levitt 2004a). This awareness—how one interacts with others—in the SPM is conceptualized as *position*.

In the beginning of treatment, the therapist tends to concentrate on teaching an approach to self-regulation and to explaining ways that therapy will be conducted. One important tool for clearly addressing the role of symptoms and the therapist's expectation(s) for therapy—especially for the client who engages in NSSI—is via a therapeutic contract (Sills 2006; Knox and Cooper 2015). The contract provides a means for identifying tolerances in therapy and setting limits. Regarding the former, the extent to which the therapy can tolerate certain behaviors needs to be specified; this sets some initial parameters for the client to self-regulate in therapy and avoids potentially confusing and distressing conversations later.

In addition to a contract, the therapist should also review the importance of learning self-care skills and ways that symptoms will be focused upon. Expectations about changing specific symptoms are also clarified and explained as is identifying and learning new approaches to managing oneself. Later, as the client's functioning improves, the therapist might guide the client to focus on more specific relationship elements.

Of course, the extent to which guided self-regulation can be accomplished is based on the degree to which the client can be open, honest, and clear about their NSSI behaviors. One can imagine that initial communications will tend to be less than direct with clients experiencing fear or shame pertaining to their NSSI behaviors or who present with enduring NSSI behaviors.

Position is a relatively simple tool that emphasizes the process of who is in charge of clients' choices and responses as well as the outcomes. Position denotes whether the client is interacting as a *victim* (i.e., things happen *to* the client and the client is unable to address the particular challenge) or a *survivor* (i.e., the client is responsible for his/her actions and is able to face the challenge). For example, a client who presents a problem as unsolvable or non-modifiable could be viewed as taking a *one-down*, passive position, whereas a client who responds with active problem solving (i.e., generating many alternatives) might be viewed as taking a *one-up position*. It could well be argued that a client who is taking a one-up position is somewhat more likely to be successful in this instance. Position is fluid in that the client can change position, learn from previous experience(s), and come at any situation from a different perspective. This underscores the import of empowering clients to be in charge of their therapy as much as possible, to make their own choices, and to see themselves as potentially effective individuals.

Position also guides how the therapist interacts with the client and provides information as to how the client may be interacting in any given situation. For example, in general interactions, the therapist observes and regularly provides feedback to the client regarding what position is being taken. In addition, the therapist regularly attends to the position that he/she is taking with the client in any particular interaction.

Position is critical in promoting a sense of self-regulation. Using the SRA, if the therapist takes a one-down position (i.e., passive, non-directive), the effect is to encourage clients to manage their own interactions and choices— to self-regulate from a survivor position (Levitt 2004a, 2004b). Thus, when the therapist defers to the client on a consistent basis, that empowers clients by communicating belief in their capability to act and to be involved in their world in a proactive manner, suggesting that clients are capable of managing themselves. In contrast, if the therapist takes a one-up position (i.e., overly directive or controlling), this tends to suggest that the therapist is encouraging dependency and potentially reinforcing a powerless, victim position.

Position is taught to clients so that they can evaluate their interactions with others, noting opportunities for changing position and potentially creating a different type of interactional outcome. Again, position is flexible and almost always under clients' general control, whether realized or not. For example, if a client approaches a particular social situation with the belief that they will "mess up" and there is nothing they could do about the situation, it is likely that they will identify areas of nonsuccess resulting in a possible sense of failure. The result is an increased likelihood of turning to NSSI to manage their emotional reaction. If, on the other hand, they recognize the position they are taking and redirect themselves to identify a more effective strategy, the probability of a more positive outcome is enhanced as is a somewhat decreased likelihood of turning to NSSI.

DEVELOPING THE THERAPEUTIC RELATIONSHIP USING THE SRA: STAGES AND ELEMENTS

As noted above, NSSI behaviors are often camouflaged by other problems such as suicidal issues, substance abuse, and eating disorders. Clients are often reluctant to disclose their NSSI behaviors because they appear to be effective at regulating mood, filling voids, finding alternatives to suicide, and so forth Getting a clear picture about the client's desire for seeking treatment can often be a challenge, and it might be difficult for the client to even disclose the NSSI behaviors at all until later in therapy development.

Clearly, an awareness of position on employing SRA is integral to developing therapeutic rapport. That is, when position is used to provide feedback and related skills to the client, the client's participation in the relationship is likely to be more proactive, involved, and enhance a desired outcome. The following outline represents an overview of the fundamental stages and elements of therapeutic relationship development using the SPM. It is presented rather briefly as a five-step process with the emphasis upon how the functions of NSSI behaviors might impact the development of the relationship and ways in which they may be communicated.

The first stage of the process is *pre-orientation*, that is, when connection is made with the therapeutic setting. Once connection between client and setting is established, the client is made aware of what therapy is and introduced to the therapist—the therapist's training, expertise, orientation, and so forth. Through the discursive process, the therapist begins to identify the "role" of the client. Hope and a positive expectations set is initiated.

The significance of pre-orientation is that the client-therapist relationship begins just as soon as any form of connection occurs and represents a therapeutic opportunity. Because many clients are reluctant to abandon NSSI behaviors, hope and a positive expectational set may be difficult to develop. It is, therefore, important that the therapist begins to convey his or her capability, knowledge, and willingness to work with NSSI and suggest that recovery is possible as soon as connection occurs. A caring, transparent rapport, along with an honest and supportive approach (one-down position) is useful for conveying belief in the client and their self-efficacy. The clinician certainly wants to reinforce the client's capacity to be proactive and successful (one-up position) in their recovery as soon as possible.

The second stage of the process is *engagement*. During this stage, the patient is further introduced to the therapist as therapy continues, expands, and deepens. Crucially, values and boundaries are clarified and legal matters such as confidentiality are discussed. The client's ability to participate in therapy is assessed, and the level of care is identified through discussion of factors such as suicidal thoughts, intent, self-harm, eating disorder behavior, OCD, anxiety, thought intrusions, substance abuse, and dissociative experiences. The SPM model is critical at this point as the client's skills and patterns of ability to initiate and sustain the *basics* is evaluated: safety, security, and physical well-being. Skills related to the *basics* are taught and monitored as appropriate.

The importance of engagement in NSSI therapy cannot be overstated. The elements of engagement above clearly identify important areas for enhancing the likelihood of the therapy and the client getting started in a positive direction. For example, clients may initially present to the therapist with verbal "understanding" of self-care behaviors, but struggle with enacting actual behavioral self-care, especially at the beginning. Therapists must pay attention to actual client behaviors, position, and follow through, regardless of the client's ability to acknowledge, understand, or verbalize what the behaviors are and/or how they can be implemented.

It is also beneficial if the therapist regularly communicates to the client that NSSI behaviors are not viewed as a personal failure or weakness and that reducing them is always the client's choice (within clinically ethical boundaries such as suicide). Engaging the client should always be about the client and their values—initially, less so about their behaviors *per se*, unless those behaviors put the client at significant risk.

During the *orientation* process, roles, vales, expectations of therapy identified are discussed, and a positive expectational set is refined, elaborated, and reinforced. Roles, skills, and behaviors of an "effective" client are described and *foundational skills* in the SPM—communication, cooperation, and collaboration—are emphasized. As the client's definition of the problem is elicited, clarified, and adopted, the therapist will develop a working "diagnosis" and impression (American Psychiatric Association 2013). Ideally, the client's expectations are openly discussed including concerns, reservations, beliefs, and/or values that could be obstacles, and the therapist/client approach to problem resolution will be reviewed openly without shame or criticism.

Orienting the client to his/her "role" can set the stage for positive expectation and outcome and reduce potential confusion about what is expected of the client in therapy, and teaching an approach to self-regulation represents the initial focus for treatment. It is vital that it is presented in a manner that the client can clearly understand and can give or deny consent. If a solid rapport that is genuine, transparent, and empowering is not in place, symptoms may be a reflection of the client's fears of the changes he or she is experiencing or a lack of confidence in the therapeutic relationship.

Alliance is developed when the problem is identified and the intent to resolve is agreed upon between client and therapist. The concept of and meaning of "change" is established from the client's viewpoint as the therapist teaches, explains, and monitors the client's ability to develop and sustain focus, direction, determination, and commitment toward resolution—that is, the *action* element of the SPM. Skills associated with task success are discussed and taught by therapist as needed by client, with client agreement and consent.

Client problem solving and alliance development are clearly intertwined. Effective problem resolution/goal attainment may enhance the alliance, and the alliance may enhance and facilitate goal achievement. If the therapist and client have been able to develop rapport, alliance development might proceed quite well; however, problems in the relationship can occur. The client might increase self-harm behaviors, switch the type of self-harming behaviors (e.g., cutting to burning) and/or add new self-harming behaviors. The client who engages in NSSI tends to communicate through their symptoms, and the alliance needs to be resilient enough to provide support for open discussion and reflection of those communications without judgment.

If the client does not embrace the problem definition and agree with the variety of selected intervention tasks or if the client does not perceive the therapeutic rapport to be safe, comforting, positive, and empathetic, the client and therapist have likely developed a therapeutic *relationship*, but not a therapeutic *alliance*. It is the elements of the therapeutic alliance that provide the safety, stability, and energy for client change that can also address residual symptoms.

Termination is not about the end of therapy. It is interconnected with therapy from the beginning. If clients have successfully moderated their self-harming behaviors to the extent to which they believe they can either remain abstinent or manage themselves without significant self-damage, successful termination proceeds relatively calmly as it would with any client.

An important point to keep in mind is that termination needs to be discussed in some manner from the start of therapy in order to avoid ruptures in the rapport which might result in an increase in self-harming. It is also essential that discussion of termination be part of the natural evolution of therapy, but it is never to be used as a threat or punishment. Within reason, the client will have some degree of control of the timing of termination.

Consequently, it is vital that the therapist be clear at the beginning as to whether he/she can work with any particular client and his or her specific symptom presentation. If there are any significant doubts, the therapist should refer to another professional as soon as possible. Of course, this must be presented to the client in a way that is not blaming or judgmental. It is very damaging to a client when the therapist becomes frustrated and refers the client out because the client is not meeting the expectations of the therapist. A perceived failure by the client can be reacted to very strongly, especially if it represents therapist rejection—no matter how it is framed. If the therapist is going to work with these clients, the therapist needs to be prepared to work with those with varying degrees of NSSI types, severity, and various other comorbid conditions for an extended period of time—often many years.

This does not mean that progress is not discussed or consultations by other member of the treatment team are not warranted and suggested. While these are, of course, essential, care must be taken not to present changes in the therapeutic rapport as representing abandonment, rejection, or due to client failure, and so forth. Hopefully, by the end of treatment, the client has learned and adopted various strategies of communication without resorting to self-harming.

THE MEANINGS OF SYMPTOMS IN SRA THERAPY

Behavioral patterns of clients who engage in NSSI communicate important information to the therapist about clients' functioning, how clients are engaging in the relationship, and so on. Using the SPM components as a backdrop for understanding, the clinician can make some general assessments about what is happening in treatment or at least what aspect of self-regulation that appears to be disrupted or impacted. Examples below represent some likely scenarios that might be experienced in NSSI treatment. For each scenario, potential areas of the SPM associated with that problem is suggested for the therapeutic team to examine, reflect upon, and possibly change.

- The client begins to exchange one behavior for another, for example, self-harm for bulimia. When this is observed, it suggests a possible disruption in sustaining the *basics*. Therapy might return to that area and explore and reestablish the patterns associated with the *basics*.
- The client begins to complain of increased trauma-related intrusions from the past. This can result in a disruption in any phase of self-regulation, reflected by interference in the continuity of the *basics, foundations skills*, or *actions*.
- The client complains that the therapist does not care as a reflection of a rupture in the therapeutic rapport or changes in the self-harm behaviors. This frequently reflects changes in management of internal information or affect(s), fears, or concerns related to perceived changes in the therapeutic relationship and/or changes in motivation. This change likely reflects a potential disruption in the areas of *foundation skills* or *actions*.
- The client demonstrates an increasing conflict with significant others. This generally reflects struggles with managing the after effects of reducing reliance upon self-harming behaviors and feeling somewhat out of control. When a client experiences these impacts, it is often demonstrated as a disruption in any of the areas of *basics, foundations skills*, or *actions*. It suggests that therapy should slow down and redirect toward the area(s) of disruption(s).
- The client begins using substances not used previously. When this occurs, the client is often struggling with the *basics* without utilizing self-harm. Their alternative skills used to sustain the *basics* may not appear to be resilient or powerful enough to the client.
- The client has been stable and progressing in recovering from self-injury behaviors, but urges to use eating disorder behaviors are increasing. This is commonly experienced when the client has been able to initially stabilize his/her self-harm behaviors, but is unsure about their efficacy or they are

responding to increased internal arousal. When explored, disruptions are often found, at least initially, in the *basics*.
- The client begins to exhibit/express strong emotions. This might suggest to the therapist that it would be beneficial to review the *basics* and reflect on the speed of introduced material related to *foundation skills*. Key initial indicators are disruption in, or problems maintaining, components of the *actions*.
- The client has learned the concepts of *position* and being a student of oneself, but these appear to be difficult for the client to apply or sustain. These types of struggles are often first suggested by disruptions in the client's *basics* and/or *foundation skills*.
- The client has done an excellent job being a student of themselves, but appears to forget how to implement previously learned skills. When this occurs, problems related to the *foundation skills* are often indicated.

DISCUSSION

In this chapter, we have briefly explored the general functions of NSSI and examined various effects those functions might have on the development and maintenance of therapeutic rapport. We have also explored various ways that NSSI might respond to and interact with the therapeutic relationship and alliance and identified some potential communication patterns and transactions often observed in the clinical arena. NSSI behaviors can present within and interact with the therapeutic relationship in various ways that are often unpredictable, threatening the therapeutic relationship/alliance and challenging the therapist to remain thoughtful, empathetic, and empowering.

It cannot be overemphasized that NSSI behaviors can impact the therapy at various stages of therapeutic relationship development. As we have seen, NSSI behaviors are used to insulate the individual from perceived strong or intolerable affects and/or connect with and relate to the therapist and others. It, therefore, goes without saying that it is important for the therapist to be acutely aware of changes in rapport as NSSI communications are often indirect and unclear.

Further, without a language to recognize, identify, and express various experiences, clients will exhibit NSSI behaviors that appear to be damaging—albeit useful in the short run. Thus, comes the following proposed caveats: First, clients may not have developed a language to identify and express their internal, or external, experiences until they learn some components of self-regulation. That is, many clients have not learned how to identify emotional experiences, how to label them relatively accurately, and how to communicate them to others effectively. The elements and skills of self-regulation learned in the context of the therapeutic relationship might help them begin to develop those tools—a language both verbal and behavioral.

Second, in addition to teaching self-regulation, and until some of the skills in the SPM are learned, the most important tasks facing therapists are to employ empathy, genuineness, tolerance, hope-building, consistent warmth, and positive regard.

Finally, it is highly recommended that therapists refrain from demanding that the client stop self-harming prior to having developed an alternative or additional repertoire of skills to communicate and self-regulate more effectively.

Clients who engage in NSSI, particularly those who have been self-harming for extended periods of time, have likely developed and integrated an approach, or methodology, to engaging in interactions or challenges based on escape and avoidance. Many clients become highly sensitive to changes in their internal system. Indeed, their arousal is easily activated, and they tend to intervene very quickly, attempting to down-regulate at any signs of arousal. In other cases, if they tend to depersonalize or "numb-out," they are quick to use NSSI to upregulate. Consequently, from a simple perspective, they are reactive to too much or too little experience and use similar behavioral approaches to address either or both conditions. Thus, NSSI behaviors serve to regulate internal experience, and therapists can be aware of the impact of changes in experience based on the degree, type, and so forth of self-harming.

Overall, the therapist needs to be able to work with the client exhibiting NSSI behaviors while facilitating and guiding the client to develop alternative skills and new methods and strategies of self-regulation and communication. This will often not be easy and will prove challenging. Ruptures in the relationship/alliance will, of course, happen, and multiple types of therapy challenges will likely occur. In the SRA, these challenges merely represent opportunities for learning and for enhanced communication. Over time, and by consistently using a SRA, most clients who engage in NSSI will learn to communicate in more effective and direct ways, relying less on the use of NSSI.

NOTES

1. Abbreviations specific to this chapter: SPM (Structural-Process Model) and SRA (Self-Regulatory Approach).

2. The Self-Regulatory Approach was developed and organized into a model of treatment—the Structural Process Model—to guide and organize treatment—discussed later in this chapter.

REFERENCES

American Psychiatric Association. *Diagnostic and Statistical Manual of Mental Disorders* (5th edition). Arlington, VA: American Psychiatric Publishing, 2013.

Andersen, Arnold E. *Practical Comprehensive Treatment of Anorexia Nervosa and Bulimia.* Baltimore: John Hopkins University Press, 1985.

Baumeister, Roy F., Todd F. Heatherton, and Dianne M. Tice. *Losing Control: How and Why People Fail at Self-Regulation.* New York: Academic Press, 1994.

Boekaerts, Monique, Paul R. Pintrich, and Moshe Zeidner. (Eds.). *Handbook of Self-Regulation.* New York: Academic Press, 2000.

Carver, Charles S., and Michael F. Scheier. *On the Self-Regulation of Behavior.* New York: Cambridge University Press, 1998.

Conterio, Karen, Wendy Lader, and Jennifer Kingston Bloom. *Bodily Harm: The Breakthrough Healing Program for Self-Injurers.* New York: Hyperion, 1998.

Endler, Norman S., and Nancy L. Kocovski. "Self-Regulation Distress in Clinical Psychology." In *Handbook of Self-Regulation*, edited by Monique Boekaerts, Paul R. Pintrich, and Moshe Zeidner, 1–9. New York: Academic Press, 2000.

Favazza, Armondo R. *Bodies Under Siege: Self-Mutilation in Culture and Psychiatry.* Baltimore: John Hopkins University Press, 1987.

Garner, David M., and L. D. Needleman. "Sequencing and Integration of Treatments." In *Handbook of Treatment for Eating Disorders* (2nd edition), edited by David M. Garner, and Paul E. Garfinkel, 50–63. New York: Guilford Press, 1997.

Haw, Camilla, Keith Hawton, Kelly Houston, and Ellen Townsend. "Psychiatric and Personality Disorders in Deliberate Self-Harm Clients." *British Journal of Psychiatry* 178, no. 1 (2001): 48–54.

Herpertz, Sabine, Henning Sass, and Armondo Favazza. "Impulsivity in Self-Mutilative Behavior: Psychometric and Biological Findings." *Journal of Psychiatric Research* 31, no. 4 (1997): 451–465.

Hsu, Lee Ann K. G. *Eating Disorders.* New York: Guildford Press, 1990.

Klonsky, E. David. "The Functions of Deliberate Self-Injury: A Review of the Evidence." *Clinical Psychology Review* 27, no. 2 (2007): 226–239.

Klonsky, E. David. "The Functions of Self-Injury in Young Adults Who Cut Themselves: Clarifying the Evidence for Affect Regulation." *Psychiatry Research* 166, no. 2–3 (2009): 260–268.

Klonsky, E. David, and Jennifer J. Muehlenkamp. "Self-Injury: A Research Review for the Practitioner." *Journal of Clinical Psychology: In Session* 63, no. 11 (2007): 1045–1056.

Klonsky, E. David, Thomas F. Oltmanns, and Eric Turkheimer. "Deliberate Self-Harm in a Nonclinical Population: Prevalence and Psychological Correlates." *American Journal of Psychiatry* 160 (2003): 1501–1508.

Knox, Rosanne, and Mick Cooper. *The Therapeutic Relationship in Counselling and Psychotherapy.* Thousand Oaks, CA: Sage Publications, Inc., 2015.

Levenkron, Steven. *Cutting: Understanding and Overcoming Self-Mutilation.* New York: W.W. Norton, 1998.

Levitt, John L. "Nature and Treatment of the Symptomatically Complex Eating Disordered Clients: Trauma, Self-Injury, and Dual Diagnosis." Invited Workshop Given at Pinecrest Christian Hospital, Professional Lecture Series, Grand Rapids, MI, March 2000a.

Levitt, John L. "Surviving the Storm: Treating the Complex Eating Disordered Client." Presented at the International Association of Eating Disorder Professional, Annual Conference, Orlando, FL, August 2000b.

Levitt, John L. "A Self-Injury and Self-Regulation: Developing a Treatment Approach." Half Day Workshop for Shelter, Inc., Northwest Community Hospital, Arlington Heights, IL, March 2001.

Levitt, John L. "A Self-Regulatory Approach to the Treatment of Eating Disorders and Self-Injury." In *Self-Harm Behavior and Eating Disorders: Dynamics, Assessment and Treatment*, edited by John L. Levitt, Randy A. Sansone, and Leigh Cohn, 211–228. New York: Brunner-Routledge, 2004a.

Levitt, John L. "Self-Regulatory Approach to Treating the Eating Disorder Patient: An Introduction." Workshop Presented to Perspectives, Chicago, August 2004b.

Levitt, John L. "A Therapeutic Approach to Treating the Eating Disorder/Borderline Personality Disorder Patient." *Eating Disorders: The Journal of Treatment and Prevention* 13, no. 1 (2005): 109–121.

Levitt, John L. "The Therapeutic Lynchpin: Managing the Relational and Emotional World of the Eating Disordered, Self-Injuring, Traumatized Client." Half Day Workshop Presented at IAEDP Symposium, Phoenix, AZ, March 2015.

Levitt, John L., and Randy A. Sansone. "Searching for the Answers: Eating Disorders and Self-Harm." *Eating Disorders: The Journal of Treatment and Prevention* 10, no. 3 (2002): 189–191.

Levitt, John L., and Randy A. Sansone. "The Treatment of Eating Disorder Clients in a Community-Based Partial Hospitalization Program." *Journal of Mental Health Counseling* 23, no. 2 (2003): 140–151.

Levitt, John L., Randy A. Sansone, and Leigh Cohn (Eds.). *Self-Harm Behavior and Eating Disorders: Dynamics, Assessment and Treatment*. New York: Brunner-Routledge, 2004.

Levitt, John L., Randy A. Sansone, and Lori A. Sansone. "Evaluating Treatment Outcomes." *Eating Disorders: The Journal of Treatment and Prevention* 11, no. 3 (2003): 241–245.

Linehan, Marsha M. *Cognitive-Behavioral Treatment of Borderline Personality Disorder*. New York: Guilford Press, 1993.

Lloyd-Richardson, Elizabeth E., Nicholas Perrine, Lisa Dierker, and Mary L. Kelley. "Characteristics and Functions of Nonsuicidal Self-Injury in a Community Sample of Adolescents." *Psychological Medicine* 37, no. 8 (2007): 1183–1192.

Miller, Dusty. *Women Who Hurt Themselves*. New York: Basic Books, 1994.

Moran, Paul, C. Coffey, Helena Romaniuk, Louisa Degenhardt, R. Borschmann, and C. George. "Substance Use in Adulthood Following Adolescent Self-Harm: A Population-Based Cohort Study." *Acta Psychiatrica Scandinavica* 131, no. 1 (2015): 61–68.

Nock, Matthew K. "Self-Injury." *Annual Review Clinical Psychology* 6 (2010): 339–363.

Sansone, Randy A., and John L. Levitt. "Self-Harm Behaviors Among Those with Eating Disorders: An Overview." *Eating Disorders: The Journal of Treatment and Prevention* 10, no. 3 (2002): 205–213.

Sansone, Randy A., and John L. Levitt. "Eating Disorders and Self-Harm: A Chaotic Intersection." *Eating Disorders Review* 14, no. 3 (2003): 1–3.

Sansone, Randy A., and Lori A. Sansone. "Assessment Tools for Self-Harm Behavior Among Those with Eating Disorders." *Eating Disorders: The Journal of Treatment and Prevention* 10, no. 3 (2002): 193–203.

Siegel, Daniel J. *The Developing Mind*. New York: Guildford Press, 1999.

Sills, Charlotte (Ed.). *Contracts in Counselling and Psychotherapy* (2nd edition). Thousand Oaks, CA: Sage.

Taylor, Peter J., Khowla Jomar, Katie Dhingra, Rebecca Forrester, Ujala Shahmalak, and Joanne M. Dickson. "A Meta-Analysis of the Prevalence of Different Functions of Non-Suicidal Self-Injury." *Journal of Affective Disorders* 227 (2018): 759–769.

Vanderlinden, Johan, and Walter Vandereycken. *Trauma, Dissociation, and Impulse Dyscontrol in Eating Disorders*. Bristol, PA: Brunner/Mazel, 1997.

Wonderlich, Stephe, Tricia Myers, Margo Norton, and Ross Crosby. "Self-Harm and Bulimia Nervosa: A Complex Connection." *Eating Disorders: The Journal of Treatment and Prevention* 10, no. 3 (2002): 257–267.

Yates, Alayne. *Compulsive Exercise and the Eating Disorders: Toward an Integrated Theory of Activity*. New York: Brunner/Mazel, 1991.

Zlotnick, Caron, Jill I. Mattia, and Mark Zimmerman. "Clinical Correlates of Self-Mutilation in a Sample of General Psychiatric Clients." *Journal of Nervous and Mental Disease* 187, no. 5 (1999): 296–301.

Chapter 3

Novel Online Daily Diary Interventions for Non-Suicidal Self-Injury
A Randomized Controlled Trial

Jill M. Hooley, Kathryn R. Fox,
Shirley B. Wang, and Anita N. D. Kwashie

INTRODUCTION

Non-suicidal self-injury (NSSI) involves intentional and self-directed harm (e.g., self-cutting, burning) that is enacted without suicidal intent (Nock 2010). Although it tends to be painful, dangerous, and stigmatized, NSSI is quite common in the general population, with lifetime prevalence rates of approximately 17 percent in adolescents and 5 percent in adults (Swannell et al. 2014). NSSI is associated with both physical and social-emotional harm in the short and long-term. A major concern is the strong link between NSSI and suicidal thoughts and behaviors both concurrently (Andover et al. 2012; Hamza et al. 2012) and prospectively (Ribeiro 2016).

All of this highlights the need for research on NSSI treatments. Unfortunately, few approaches to date have consistently reduced NSSI compared to active control treatments (Brausch and Girresch 2012; Glenn et al. 2015; Gonzales and Bergstrom 2013; Washburn et al. 2012). One notable exception is the intervention developed by Franklin et al. (2016). This intervention, called Therapeutic Evaluative Conditioning (TEC), uses a form of Pavlovian conditioning (Hofmann et al. 2010) to *increase* aversion to self-injury stimuli (e.g., knives, blood) and to *decrease* aversion to the self (i.e., reduce self-criticism). Utilizing an online, app-based treatment and across three randomized control trials, TEC resulted in significant reductions in NSSI, suicide plans, and suicide attempts, compared to an active control treatment.

Franklin et al.'s (2016) approach is notable for three primary reasons. First, it targeted two relatively novel treatment targets for NSSI based on growing evidence that high self-criticism and low aversion to NSSI stimuli are important NSSI risk factors (Hooley and Franklin 2018). Second, TEC reduced both NSSI and suicidal thoughts and behaviors, suggesting that these treatment targets may prove effective for a range of self-injurious thoughts and behaviors. Third, TEC was the first highly scalable, inexpensive, online treatment to be developed for NSSI. Results from Franklin et al.'s (2016) study demonstrated that (a) targeting new risk factors such as self-criticism and diminished aversion to NSSI stimuli may be effective for reducing NSSI and (b) that it is possible to conduct online treatments for NSSI.

In the present study, we sought to use this information to create a new, online treatment program for NSSI. Specifically, we conducted a randomized controlled trial (RCT) to evaluate Autobiographical Self-Enhancement Training (ASET)—a novel, cognitive intervention for NSSI focused on reducing self-criticism and enhancing positive self-worth. To help reduce NSSI engagement, self-worth was selected as a primary treatment target for several reasons. First, people who engage in NSSI demonstrate lowered levels of self-worth across several domains, including body image (Muehlenkamp and Brausch 2012), self-dissatisfaction (Victor and Klonsky 2014), and self-criticism (Glassman et al. 2007; Hooley et al. 2010). Second, recent longitudinal research found that implicit and explicit self-criticism predicted continued NSSI engagement over a four-week follow-up period above and beyond other relevant factors (Fox et al. 2017), suggesting that self-criticism may be an important NSSI risk factor and potential treatment target. Third, experimental research has demonstrated that pain endurance is elevated among people who engage in NSSI and that reducing self-criticism normalizes this (Hooley and St. Germain 2014). Finally, as noted above, a recent treatment study designed to reduce self-criticism as well as increase aversion to NSSI stimuli decreased NSSI engagement over the treatment period (Franklin et al. 2016). Given this compelling body of research implicating self-criticism as an important NSSI risk factor, we hypothesized that decreasing self-criticism would result in lowered rates of NSSI engagement when compared to treatments targeting other factors. However, unlike the approach adopted by Franklin and colleagues which involved conditioning, we used a more explicit method in an effort to target self-criticism more directly and in a manner that involved participants' awareness, perhaps, therefore, improving treatment effects.

For the present RCT, we tested ASET against another potentially active treatment (expressive writing [EW]) and also against a control treatment (journaling). The ASET intervention was based on a cognitive intervention previously used for participants with NSSI histories. Specifically, Hooley and St. Germain (2014) created a brief intervention that, during one in-lab session, significantly increased positive self-worth and decreased the amount of time participants were willing to endure pain compared to two comparison conditions. ASET was designed to test whether a similar cognitive intervention, administered online, would decrease self-criticism over time and to test whether these decreases would extend to subsequent decreases in NSSI compared to alternative interventions.

We also tested an intervention that involved EW. EW, a procedure first developed by Pennebaker and Beall (1986) involves writing about stressful or upsetting experiences. Many years of research have established that EW produces psychological and physical health benefits (Smyth 1998). Although NSSI is used to regulate negative emotions (Hooley and Franklin 2018), to date, no study has examined EW as an intervention for NSSI. Finally, we used a journaling (JNL) condition as a comparison control intervention. This involved writing about daily events without any focus on emotional issues. The JNL intervention was developed to control for daily writing (which was integral to both the ASET and the EW conditions).

We predicted that, compared to the control (JNL) condition, ASET treatment would significantly reduce self-criticism, NSSI, and the desire to engage in NSSI. Depressive symptoms were included as a secondary treatment target because there is high comorbidity between depressive symptoms and NSSI (Nock et al. 2010). Meta-analytic evidence further suggests that self-esteem (related to self-criticism) longitudinally predicts depression (Sowislo and Orth 2013). Similarly, because NSSI tends to be comorbid with suicidal thoughts and behaviors (Andover et al. 2012; Hamza et al. 2012), these were also selected as secondary treatment targets. We hypothesized that ASET would reduce depressive symptoms, suicidal thoughts, and suicidal behaviors compared to JNL. We also predicted that compared to the JNL condition, EW would provide general benefits and reduce feelings of depression. However, because EW does not target self-criticism, we did not predict that participants assigned to this condition would show significant decreases in self-criticism, desire to self-injure and engage in NSSI, or engagement in suicidal thoughts and behaviors.

METHOD

Recruitment and Participants

This study was conducted in accordance with the Declaration of Helsinki. All study components were approved by the Institutional Review Board at Harvard University and all participants provided informed consent. Adopting the method used by Franklin and colleagues (Franklin et al. 2016), participants were recruited from online forums related to self-injury and severe psychopathology (e.g., reddit.com/r/depression). Research increasingly supports the use of online methods for valid collection of data and shows that online and in-person studies result in similar outcomes across tasks and populations. Such an approach is particularly useful when studying stigmatized or taboo topics, like self-injury. This is because online study assessment allows for greater participant anonymity and privacy, potentially increasing participant comfort in disclosing stigmatized thoughts, behaviors, and symptoms, including self-injury.

After determining eligibility via a screening questionnaire (i.e., 18+ years of age, daily Internet access, English fluency, and 2+ episodes of NSSI in the past month), forum members interested in participating completed an online consent form and an approximately 45-minute baseline assessment. Eight participants tried to enter the study multiple times or did not answer the majority (i.e., 90%+) of the baseline assessment questions, indicating problems with validity. These participants were excluded. All participants were entered into the study between July 2016 and September 2016. Figure 3.1 summarizes the flow of recruitment.

The final sample included 144 adults (85.40% female) aged eighteen to forty-five years (M_{age} = 25.63, SD = 5.83) who reported two or more past month NSSI episodes. Most participants lived in the United States (71.53%) and identified as Caucasian (87.50%), with remaining participants identifying as Black (2.08%), Hispanic (2.08%), Asian (3.69%), Native American (3.47%), or Other (3.47%). Additionally, the majority of participants endorsed lifetime (83.33%) and past month psychiatric treatment (52.08%), and many were currently using psychiatric medications (45.83%).

Treatment Conditions

After completion of the baseline assessment, participants were randomly assigned to one of three treatment groups: JNL (N = 46), EW (N = 49), and ASET (N = 49) using randomization software within Qualtrics. Each treatment condition was designed as a brief, daily diary treatment that could be completed from home or from a mobile device anywhere with Internet access. Participants assigned to the ASET condition were asked to write for five minutes each day about something that happened that day that made them feel good about themselves as a person. Participants assigned to the EW condition were asked to write for five minutes each day about something that bothered them or was on their mind that day. Participants in the JNL condition were asked to write for five minutes each day about the events of the day in a general and factually descriptive way (see table 3.1 for full directions and table 3.2 for examples of writing relevant to each condition). For all conditions, writing responses were monitored daily.

Participants were asked to complete daily writing assignments as well as brief weekly assessments during the treatment month (i.e., twenty-eight days).

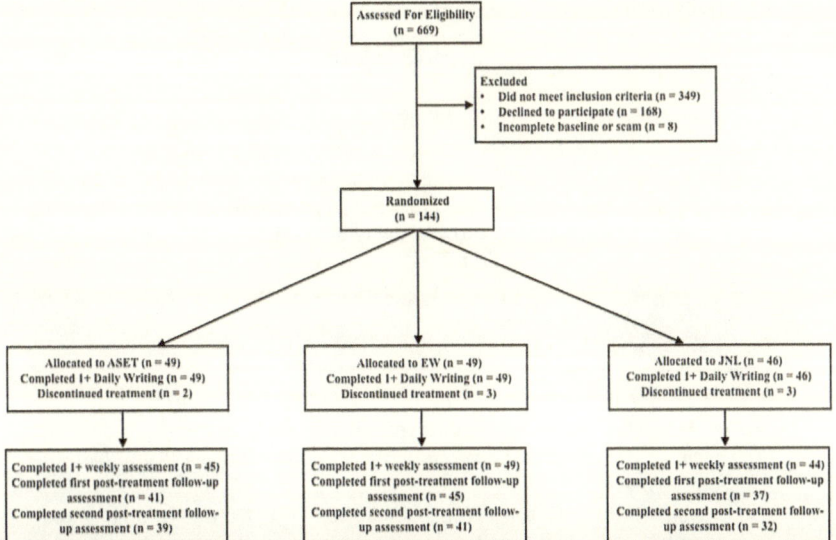

Figure 3.1 CONSORT Diagram Illustrating Flow through the Various Stages of the Study. *Source*: Author Created.

Four weeks after the end of treatment, participants were contacted again (i.e., one-month follow up; eight weeks after baseline; $N = 123$ (85.42%) to complete the first follow-up assessment. A second and final follow up occurred eight weeks later (i.e., three-month follow-up; sixteen weeks after baseline; $N = 118$ (82.64%).

To maintain participant anonymity, participants were asked to use an email address without identifiable information (e.g., their date of birth or legal name). During the writing phase of the study, participants were emailed daily at 4:00 p.m. (adjusted to their time zone) with a reminder to complete the daily writing assignment. They were also provided with a link to Qualtrics to complete this assignment. Participants were compensated at the end of each week via Amazon, Starbucks, or iTunes gift cards. Participants were compensated $10 for completing the baseline assessment, $2 for each daily writing they completed, $5 for each weekly assessment completed during the treatment month, and $20 for each follow-up assessment completed. To increase participant engagement in the active treatment phase, participants were given a $24 bonus for completing at least 26/28 of the daily writing assignments in addition to each weekly assessment. Additionally, participants who completed at least 20/28 daily writing assignments were entered into a drawing for one of ten $50 gift cards.

The integrity of the treatment was monitored daily. If participants did not submit their daily writing by 2:00 a.m. (personalized to their time zone) or if they submitted a response that did not follow the instructions for their assigned

Table 3.1 Daily Writing Directions

Group	Directions
ASET	Now we'd like you to think about a specific positive characteristic you showed *today*. It doesn't have to be a big thing— small things count too! Opening a door open for someone, for instance, is a good example of thoughtfulness. Think back and come up with a specific example. Were you kind, or loyal, or funny? How about being a good friend or a good listener? So long as it is a positive characteristic you showed today, it counts! On the next screen, we would like you to spend around five minutes writing about the positive event you just thought about. As you write try and be as specific as you can and tell us: • What happened? • How did you feel? • Was anyone else involved? If so, how do you think they felt? • Are there other examples of times you showed these qualities? The focus of your writing should be on what you did that made you feel good about yourself. All of your writing is COMPLETELY CONFIDENTIAL. No one is judging you. And don't worry about spelling, sentence structure, or grammar. The only rule is that once you begin writing, you write continuously for about five minutes.
EW	Now we'd like you to think about something that has been on your mind or has concerned or worried you *today*. On the next screen, we would like you to write for around five minutes about a moment from *TODAY* that's been on your mind or bothered you in some way. Just use this opportunity to explore your emotions and thoughts about your chosen moment. You might write about: • Anything stressful you're currently experiencing • Your relationships with others, including parents, lovers, friends, or relatives • Anything concerning your past, your present, or your future • Who you have been, who you would like to be, or who you are now The focus of your writing should be on your emotions and thoughts about anything from today. All of your writing is COMPLETELY CONFIDENTIAL. No one is judging you. And don't worry about spelling, sentence structure, or grammar. The only rule is that once you begin writing, you write continuously for about 5 minutes.
JNL	Now we'd like you to think about how you spent your time *today*. On the next screen, we would like you to write for 5 minutes about how you spent your time *TODAY*. Do NOT include any emotions, feelings or opinions in your writing. Instead, we'd like for you to write in a factual, descriptive way. The focus of your writing should be on the factual aspects of your day's events and activities. All of your writing is COMPLETELY CONFIDENTIAL. No one is judging you. And don't worry about spelling, sentence structure, or grammar. The only rule is that once you begin writing, you write continuously for about 5 minutes.

Source: Author Created.

Table 3.2 Examples of Daily Writing

ASET	So I was helpful today! Today I was going into my apartment and I saw my neighbor struggling to get her luggage up the stairs. She's a bit older and it looked like she was struggling with the weight, so I asked her if she'd like some help. She said yes, so I carried her luggage all the way up to the third floor. It felt good to help her out because she looked kind of frail, and she was really sweet and grateful. We chatted a bit after about her life, and I liked talking to her. I think she enjoyed talking to me too. I was glad that I was able to make her day a little easier.
EW	Graduation is coming up fast, and I'm really stressed out about what I'm going to do when college is over. I feel as if everyone already has a job lined up, and I've still got nothing. And so many of my friends are leaving for graduate school. It's like everyone has the next stages of their lives figured out, and I'm stuck. Should I move back home with my parents? Or maybe live somewhere cheap and work a couple of minimum wage jobs until something works out? There are so many options, but I don't actually know which one to take.
JNL	I woke up at 11:00 a.m. and I took a shower and washed my hair. I got dressed and made my breakfast. I had a bowl of cereal, a banana, and a coffee. Then I got in my car and drove to the office where I work. When I got to work, I answered five emails and went to a meeting. The meeting took until 12:30 p.m. I went to a nearby restaurant to buy some lunch. I came back to work and sent more emails. I took a break to talk with my work friends. After work I went to the gym and I ran on the treadmill. Then I drove home. I ordered takeout from a nearby Chinese restaurant and browsed the internet. Then I ate my takeout and called my parents. Then I called my friend to make plans for the weekend.

Source: Author Created

condition (e.g., they included emotional content in the JNL condition), a study coordinator emailed them to remind them to complete the writing assignments daily, to remind them of the compensation structure of the study, and/or to remind them to follow the study guidelines in their writing. Not including missed responses—0.02 percent, 5.38 percent, and 7.04 percent of daily writings in the EW, JNL, and ASET conditions respectively—prompted experimenter emails. These were sent primarily because responses were too short (all three conditions), they did not include the requisite focus on doing something positive or contained too much overall negative content (ASET condition only), or they included emotional content (JNL condition only).

Measures

Demographic Information. We assessed basic demographic information including age, sex, gender, and race. Additionally, we assessed lifetime and past month use of psychiatric treatment as well as current use of psychiatric medications.

Modified Self-Injurious Thoughts and Behaviors Interview (SITBI; Nock et al. 2007). The SITBI is typically a semi-structured interview used to assess the presence, frequency, and characteristics of self-injurious thoughts and behaviors, including suicidal and non-suicidal self-injury. The interview has strong interrater reliability (average $\kappa = .99$) and strong convergent and construct validity, indexed by its association with other measures of self-injurious thoughts and behaviors. As with other online research studies (Fox et al. 2016; Franklin et al. 2016), we used an online version of the SITBI to assess history of self-injurious thoughts and behaviors. Prior research suggests that online and in-person versions of the SITBI produce similar estimates (Franklin et al. 2014).

In addition to questions assessing lifetime history and frequency of self-injurious thoughts and behaviors, the SITBI was used to asses self-reported desire to discontinue and likelihood of future NSSI from 0 (not at all) to 4 (extremely).

Beck Depression Inventory—II (BDI-II; Beck et al. 1996). The BDI-II is a twenty-one-item self-report questionnaire assessing symptoms of depression. All items are rated on a four-point scale. Higher scores on the BDI-II index more severe depressive symptoms. The BDI-II demonstrates high internal consistency and strong convergent and discriminant validity among psychiatric outpatients (Steer et al. 1999). Cronbach's alpha for the BDI-II was excellent, ranging from .92 to .96 at all-time points.

Self-Rating Scale (SRS; Hooley et al. 2010). The SRS is an eight-item measure that assesses self-critical cognitions (e.g., "I often feel inferior to others," "I am socially inept and socially undesirable"). Items are answered on a seven-point Likert scale, ranging from strongly disagree to strongly agree, with higher scores indexing higher levels of self-criticism. The SRS demonstrates good internal reliability and can differentiate groups with and without NSSI histories (ibid.; St. Germain and Hooley 2011). Cronbach's alpha for this measure was high and ranged from .84 to .94 at all assessments.

Post Study Assessment. During the final follow-up assessment, participants were questioned about the acceptability of the treatment they received. Specifically, they were asked to respond to the following statements using a scale from 1 (strongly disagree) to 7 (strongly agree): "I enjoyed writing each day," "I found the writing task annoying," "I didn't understand why I was doing the writing task," "I plan to keep writing each day because I found it really helpful."

Data Analytic Plan

Retention and Missing Data. Retention rates were calculated for each week during the treatment month and at the end of the one-month and three-month post-treatment follow ups. There were no significant treatment group differences in retention rates across any of these assessment points. Missing data were minimal (7.1%) and did not differ across treatment groups ($p > .05$).

Outcomes. Primary outcomes were NSSI episodes and self-criticism. We also examined the effects of treatment on depression, desire to discontinue NSSI, likelihood of future NSSI, days of active suicide ideation, and days of suicide plans.

Statistical Models. We utilized mixed-effects regression models for between-group analyses examining the effect of treatment group on outcomes at the end of treatment and post-treatment follow-up assessments. These models allow for inclusion of participants with missing data; therefore, all participants who completed baseline assessments and at least one end-of-treatment or post-treatment assessment were included in analyses.

All mixed effects models included an interaction term between treatment group and assessment time point as fixed effects and a random intercept for each participant. Additionally, all models controlled for baseline levels of the outcome variable. We fit linear mixed-effects models using the R package lmerTest (Kuznetsova et al. 2016) for continuous outcome measures (self-criticism, depression, desire to discontinue NSSI, likelihood of future NSSI). NSSI episodes, days of active suicide ideation, and days of suicide plans are count variables that tend to be positively skewed and include an excess of zeros. Accordingly, we fit zero-inflated negative binomial mixed-effects models using the R package glmmTMB (Magnusson 2017) for these outcome variables.

Pairwise comparisons between treatment groups at all assessment points (end of treatment, post-treatment follow-up assessments one and two) were assessed with the R package lsmeans (Lenth and Hervé 2015). To examine overall clinical change (regardless of treatment group) from baseline to the end of treatment, we conducted paired samples t-tests for all outcome variables using SPSS.

Overview of Treatment-Related Analyses. We were primarily interested in the overall effects of treatment group (ASET vs. EW vs. JNL). Therefore, resembling intention-to-treat tests, our analyses included all participants who completed baseline assessments, were randomized to a treatment group, and completed at least one other assessment at any time point, regardless of whether they completed all daily writings. Although treatment participation differed across treatment groups, as reported below, there were no significant differences in retention rates for assessments between groups. Controlling for the number of completed daily writings also did not change our findings in any important ways. Similarly, with the exception of self-criticism (see endnote 1), controlling for baseline differences in depression did not change results in any way.

Treatment and Follow-Up Analyses. We sought to examine whether treatment group significantly predicted self-criticism, depression, and self-injurious thoughts and behavior variables (including NSSI and suicidal thoughts and behaviors) at the end of the treatment month, as well as whether these effects were maintained after treatment ended. Therefore, we used an interaction term to test the effects of treatment group across three time points (end of treatment, one-month post-treatment follow-up and three-month post-treatment follow-up). All analyses control for baseline levels of the relevant outcome variable by using baseline scores as a covariate in the model.

Suicidal Behavior Analyses. Suicidal behavior is a low base rate behavior, especially across short time periods. Thus, as with other similar treatment studies (Franklin et al. 2016), we calculated a suicidal behavior variable that included all behaviors throughout the treatment month and at post-treatment follow-up assessments. Because this variable was calculated as the sum of all suicidal behaviors across all time points, we fit a model with treatment group as a single predictor variable, rather than as an interaction term with assessment time point. The zero-inflated portion of the model was also specified with this fixed effect.

RESULTS

There were no significant demographic or psychiatric treatment history differences among the three groups (all $ps > .05$). Additionally, there were no group differences in self-criticism at baseline ($p = .34$), or in self-reported episodes of past week, month, or year NSSI, suicide ideation, suicide plans, or suicide attempts (all $ps > .05$). However, there were significant differences in baseline depression ($F(2) = 3.70$, $p = .03$). Probing these differences in more detail, Bonferroni corrected post-hoc tests indicated that participants in the ASET condition had significantly lower depression scores than participants in the EW ($p = .04$), but not the JNL condition at baseline; no other group differences were statistically significant. Means for all baseline measures are provided in table 3.3.

Treatment Participation. All participants completed at least one daily writing assignment. Most participants (77.08%) completed more than twenty-one daily writings with similar proportions across groups (ASET group: 67.35%, EW group: 83.67%, JNL group: 80.43%). However, groups differed significantly in the total number of daily writings completed ($F(2) = 3.69$, $p = .03$). Bonferroni corrected post-hoc tests revealed that participants completed significantly more daily writing assignments in the EW condition ($M = 23.65$; $SD = 5.18$) compared to the ASET condition ($M = 21.31$, $SD = 7.36$; $p < .05$). There were no significant differences in the number of daily writings completed by participants in any other condition.

Retention Rates for Follow-Up Assessments. Retention rates gradually dropped or remained stable from treatment week one to treatment week four (i.e., 95.14%, 92.36%, 86.81%, 87.50%, respectively). A total of 95.83

Table 3.3 Baseline Scores for Clinical Measures

	ASET (n = 49) M(SD)	EW (n = 49) M(SD)	JNL (n = 46) M(SD)
Self-criticism	43.59(8.93)[a]	44.73(7.61)[a]	42.07(9.60)[a]
Depression	33.04(14.53)[a]	40.06(13.65)[b]	39.29(13.30)[b]
Self-cutting episodes	2.33(3.04)[a]	4.02(6.82)[a]	2.89(7.21)[a]
Overall NSSI episodes	7.20(8.30)[a]	10.22(12.26)[a]	9.59(13.47)[a]
Desire to discontinue NSSI	2.29(0.95)[a]	2.12(1.21)[a]	2.27(1.31)[a]
Likelihood of future NSSI	3.06(1.08)[a]	3.15(1.04)[a]	3.00(0.98)[a]
Suicide ideation	9.00(10.53)[a]	10.63(10.89)[a]	12.98(11.49)[a]
Suicide plans	4.96(8.42)[a]	4.02(7.32)[a]	5.57(7.76)[a]
Suicidal behaviors	0.45(1.68)[a]	0.16(0.55)[a]	0.33(0.76)[a]

Note. ASET = Autobiographical Self-Enhancement Training; EW = Expressive Writing; JNL = Journaling. Means with different subscripts are significantly different at $p < .05$ from other means within the same row.
Source; Author Created.

percent of participants completed at least one of the weekly assessments during the treatment month and 81.25 percent of participants completed all follow-ups, with no differences in completion rates among groups. During post-treatment months, retention rates remained relatively stable across follow-up assessments at one-month (85.42%) and three-months post-treatment (82.64%), again with no differences across treatment groups.

Overall Clinical Change

Regardless of treatment group, participants demonstrated significant reductions in self-criticism ($t(125) = 3.69$, $p < .001$) and overall NSSI episodes ($t(125) = 2.38$, $p = .02$) from baseline to the end of treatment. These findings are illustrated in figures 3.2 and 3.3. There were also significant decreases in depression ($t(122) = 7.91$, $p < .001$) and suicide ideation ($t(121) = 2.41$, $p = .02$) over this same period. Desire to discontinue NSSI, likelihood of future NSSI, or suicide plans, or suicidal behaviors remained unchanged.

Treatment Analyses

Self-Criticism.[1] The ASET group reported significantly less self-criticism at the end of treatment than the JNL group ($B = -4.31$, $SE = 1.81$, $p = .047$), but not the EW group ($p = .16$). However, this effect was not maintained through either the first ($p = .46$) or second ($p = .41$) post-treatment follow-up assessment.

Depression. No significant effects of treatment group were detected for depression at the end of treatment or post-treatment follow-up assessments.

Overall NSSI Episodes. No significant effects of treatment group were detected for overall NSSI episodes at the end of treatment or at the one- or three-month follow-up assessments.

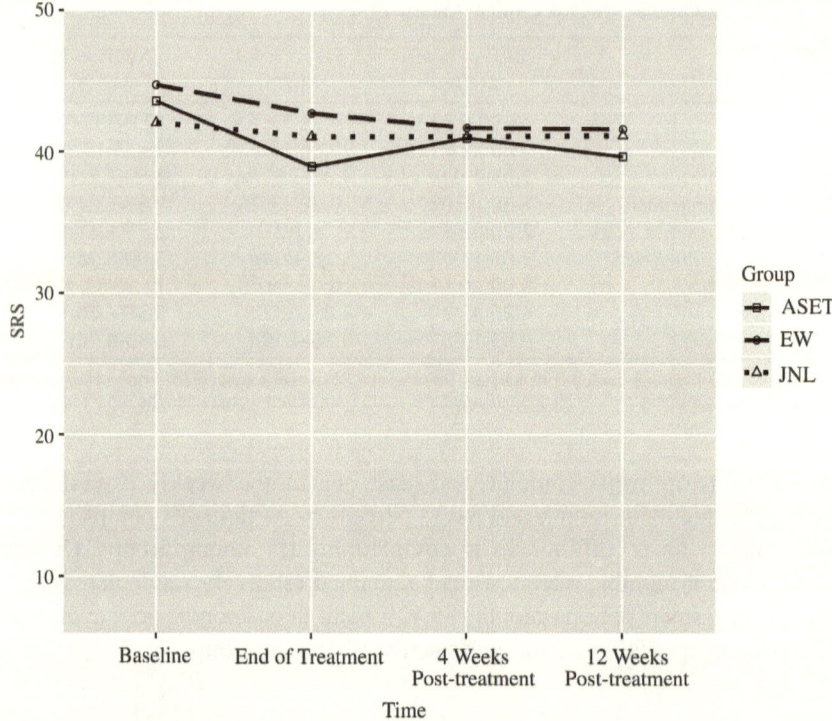

Figure 3.2 Self-criticism by treatment group. The ASET group reported significantly less self-criticism at the end of treatment than the JNL group ($p = .047$), but not the EW group ($p = .16$). However, this effect was not maintained through either the first ($p = .46$) or second ($p = .41$) post-treatment follow-up assessment. *Source*: Author Created.

Desire to Discontinue NSSI. No significant effects of treatment group were detected for desire to discontinue NSSI at the end of treatment or at the follow-up assessments.

Likelihood of Future NSSI. No significant effects of treatment group were detected for likelihood of future NSSI at the end of treatment or at the follow-up assessments.

Suicide Ideation. The JNL group reported significantly fewer days of suicide ideation than the EW group (but not the ASET group) at the end of treatment ($B = -0.62$, $SE = 0.26$, $p = .04$); this effect did not reach significance at the one-month post-treatment follow-up assessment ($p = .33$), but was maintained at the three-month follow-up assessment ($B = -0.57$, $SE = 0.19$, $p = .001$). There was also a trend toward the ASET group reporting significantly fewer days of suicide ideation at the end of treatment compared with the EW group ($B = -0.60$, $SE = 0.27$, $p = .07$). This did not reach significance at the one-month post-treatment follow-up assessment ($p = .52$), but was apparent

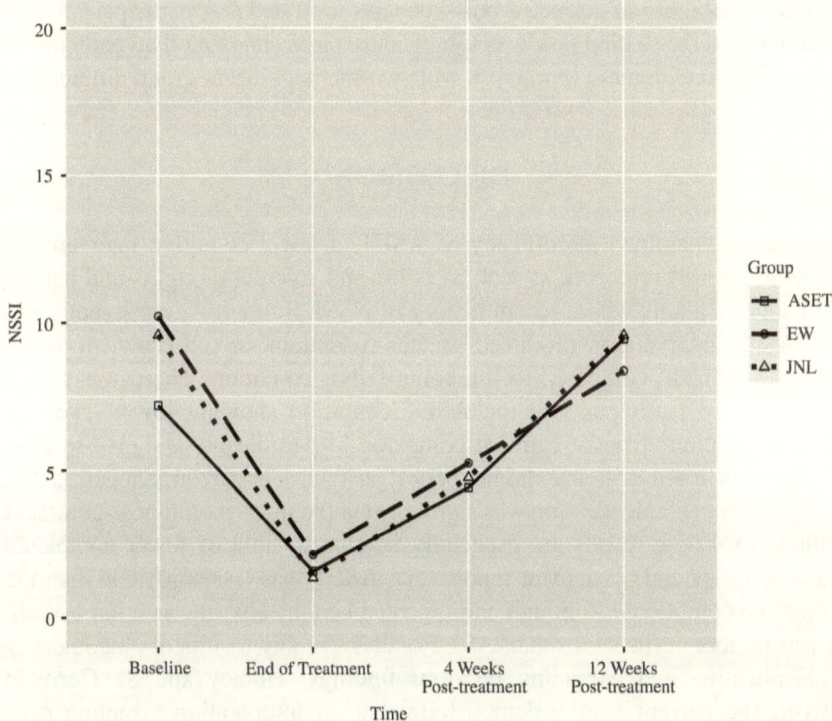

Figure 3.3 **NSSI episodes by treatment group.** There was a significant reduction in NSSI from baseline to the end of treatment ($p = .02$), but no significant effects of treatment group at the end of treatment or at post-treatment follow-ups. *Source*: Author Created.

at the three-month post-treatment follow-up assessment ($B = -0.50$, $SE = 0.21$, $p = .048$).

Suicide Plans. No significant effects of treatment group were detected for suicide plans at the end of treatment or post-treatment follow-up assessments.

Suicidal Behaviors. No significant effects of treatment group were detected for suicidal behaviors throughout the treatment month or post-treatment follow-up assessments.

Acceptability of Treatment. There were no significant group differences in self-reported understanding of the reason for completing daily writing assignments, or for self-reported helpfulness of the daily writing assignment ($ps = .10$ and .64 respectively). However, there were significant group differences in finding the writing task enjoyable ($F(2) = 5.55$, $p = .01$) and finding the writing task annoying ($F(2) = 3.10$, $p = .05$). Bonferroni corrected post-hoc tests indicated that participants in the ASET condition found the daily writing task to be significantly less enjoyable than participants than the EW condition ($p = .01$) but not the JNL condition, though effects were trending toward significance ($p = .07$).

Similarly, Bonferroni corrected post-hoc tests indicated that participants in the ASET found the writing task was significantly more annoying than participants in the EW condition did ($p = .047$), with no other significant group differences.

DISCUSSION

This study examined the efficacy of ASET, a novel cognitive intervention, in reducing self-criticism, as well as NSSI and suicidal thoughts and behaviors, among adults with a recent history of NSSI. Supporting our hypotheses, the ASET intervention produced greater reductions in self-criticism at the end of treatment compared to the control JNL condition. There was also a trend toward participants in the ASET condition showing lower levels of suicide ideation at post-treatment compared to participants assigned to EW. Reductions in self-criticism did not persist past the active treatment period, but the effect for suicide ideation was significant at the three-month post-treatment follow-up. These results are especially notable in light of fewer completed daily writings and participant reports that ASET was less enjoyable than the other two conditions. Although participants liked the EW intervention overall, it was no more efficacious than ASET or JNL for any treatment outcome.

Replicating and extending previous findings (Hooley and St. Germain 2014), the current results demonstrate that an intervention targeting self-criticism decreases both self-criticism and suicide ideation among individuals with NSSI. It also warrants mention that, overall, all of our writing-based approaches provided clinical benefits and reduced episodes of NSSI. Given the high prevalence of NSSI behaviors in clinical and nonclinical populations (Swannell et al. 2014; Selby et al. 2012) as well as their concerning associations with suicide (Ribeiro 2016), highly scalable and disseminable treatments are needed to reduce these dangerous behaviors. These findings provide further evidence supporting the feasibility and acceptability of online interventions for NSSI.

Although these results are promising, they should be interpreted with caution. Despite significant reductions in self-criticism following the ASET intervention, levels of self-criticism continued to remain quite high for individuals in all treatment groups and reductions did not persist after treatment termination. Moreover, many clinical outcomes remained unchanged, such that no treatment was significantly more successful than the others in reducing overall NSSI episodes, suicide plans, suicidal behaviors, depression, desire to discontinue NSSI, or likelihood of engaging in future NSSI.

The finding that the JNL treatment reduced suicide ideation compared to EW was unexpected and warrants consideration. It is also interesting in light of recent findings from another RCT. Celano et al. (2017) compared a positive psychology-based intervention with a cognition-focused control intervention among high-risk patients discharged from inpatient care. The cognition-focused intervention, which had some similarities to our JNL intervention, required participants to recount three events occurring each day, in an emotionally neutral manner, for the duration of treatment. Contrary to expectation, the cognition-focused intervention resulted in significantly larger reductions in hopelessness at the six-week follow-up, and significant reductions in depression and suicidality at both six and twelve week follow-up assessments. Results suggest that encouraging people who may be at high risk for self-injurious thoughts and behaviors to think about their days in the absence of emotional content could be palliative. However, it is important to keep in mind that the JNL condition did not outperform EW or ASET in reducing NSSI episodes or other self-injury outcomes. Additional studies are needed to more fully evaluate the potential benefits of writing about the events of one's day in a nonemotional manner.

Findings for the current study should also be considered in the context of the study's limitations. First, participants were predominantly white and female young adults who were recruited from online forums related to self-injury and psychopathology. It is, therefore, unclear whether these findings would generalize to individuals of other ages, ethnicities, or genders recruited in other ways. All outcome data were also based on self-report. This is not unusual for studies of this type, as participant anonymity helps decrease the potential for demand characteristics. Nonetheless we acknowledge this as a limitation. The fact that participants were paid for their participation may also have impacted their willingness and motivation to complete the daily writing assignments and our moderate sample sizes may have precluded our ability to detect all but the largest treatment effects on clinical outcomes. Finally, all participants completed standard, once-daily, 5-minute writing assignments. It is possible that higher dosages of each treatment (e.g., greater number of writing assignments per day; longer length of writing assignments) would produce greater reductions in self-criticism and self-injurious thoughts and behaviors.

One unexpected finding from the current study was that all participants improved over the course of treatment, regardless of the treatment condition to which they were assigned. In other words, all forms of daily writing were helpful. More specifically, all approaches reduced episodes of NSSI, self-criticism, depression, and suicide ideation. This could reflect regression to the mean, although improvement was not noted across all outcome variables. Another nonspecific factor that should be considered is participants' knowledge that members of the research team were paying attention to them and reading their daily writings. This sense of connection, however, temporary, may have been helpful. Future studies involving journaling would do well to consider the possibility that this may be a more active treatment approach than might be apparent at first glance. With hindsight, it would have been advantageous to also include another comparison group that received no online intervention whatsoever, or one in which participants were receiving equivalent contact with researchers. This would have allowed us to determine more about whether the simple act of journaling in an emotionally neutral manner is beneficial for individuals with NSSI.

Overall, this study contributes important new information about the feasibility and efficacy of novel online interventions for NSSI. Findings further suggest that although self-criticism may be an important treatment target in NSSI, altering self-criticism appears to be particularly difficult for individuals with severe and recent NSSI histories and high levels of depression. People who engage in NSSI do not appear to like focusing on their positive attributes. This may be because their negative beliefs about the self are well established and entrenched. It is possible that more direct (one-on-one) approaches are needed to provide additional direction and support for overcoming the cognitive challenges presented by considering alternative and more positive aspects of their identities. Alternatively, more covert or implicit approaches capable of enhancing positive self-concept without triggering resistance could be considered. In contrast, writing about negative emotions, such as occurred in the EW condition, appears to be much more enjoyable for people who engage in NSSI. One reassuring aspect of our data is the finding that such a focus on negative emotions in the context of EW does not increase the likelihood of negative outcomes. This seems important to know.

CONCLUSION

Future research should examine the effects of ASET on self-criticism and self-injurious thoughts and behaviors among individuals with less severe clinical presentations. The potential for online interventions such as the one described here to prevent the development of NSSI should also be considered. Adolescence is a time of increased self-criticism and increased risk for NSSI. Interventions that focus attention on positive self-attributes may provide some protection against the development of NSSI. Further research is also needed to test the benefits of ASET as an adjunct to existing treatments, in addition to a stand-alone intervention. Although much remains to be learned, the current findings demonstrate that ASET is a feasible and potentially promising intervention that is cost effective, easily accessible, and highly scalable. The benefits of non-emotional journaling also warrant increased consideration.

DECLARATIONS

Ethics Approval and Consent to Participate

This study was reviewed and approved by the Harvard University Committee on the Use of Humans Subjects. All participants provided written informed consent.

Consent for Publication

Not applicable.

Availability of Data and Material

The datasets generated and analyzed for the current study are not publicly available due to confidentiality concerns but are available from the corresponding author on reasonable request.

Competing Interests

None of the authors report any competing interests.

Funding

This research was supported by a grant from the Eric M. Mindich Research Fund for the Foundations of Human Behavior to Jill M. Hooley

Authors' Contributions

JMH and KRF designed the study and JMH secured funding. KRF and ANK were responsible for data collection and SBW and KRF conducted statistical analysis under supervision from JMH. All authors were involved in drafting the manuscript and all authors approved the final submission.

Acknowledgments

We thank Summer Peterson and Olga Revzina for their assistance with data collection.

NOTE

1. When controlling for baseline depression, the stronger effect of ASET than JNL in reducing self-criticism at the end of treatment was no longer significant ($p = .11$); however, ASET and JNL did not significantly differ in depression at baseline, and depression did not have a significant main effect ($p = .22$).

REFERENCES

Andover, Margaret S., Blair W. Morris, Abigail Wren, and Margaux E. Bruzzese. "The Co-Occurrence of Non-Suicidal Self-Injury and Attempted Suicide Among Adolescents: Distinguishing Risk Factors and Psychosocial Correlates." *Child and Adolescent Psychiatry and Mental Health* 6, no. 11 (2012). doi: 10.1186/1753-2000-6-11.

Beck, Aaron T., Robert A. Steer, and Gregory K. Brown. *Beck Depression Inventory-II*. San Antonio, TX: Psychological Corporation, 1996: 12–15. doi: 10.1037/t00742-000.

Brausch, Amy M., and Sarah K. Girresch. "A Review of Empirical Treatment Studies for Adolescent Nonsuicidal Self-Injury." *Journal of Cognitive Psychotherapy* 26 (2012): 3–18. doi: 10.1891/0889-8391.26.1.3.

Celano, C. M., E. E. Beale, C. A. Mastromauro, J. G. Stewart, R. A. Millstein, R. P. Auerbach, C. A. Bedoya, and J. C. Huffman. "Psychological Interventions to Reduce Suicidality in High-Risk Patients with Major Depression: A Randomized Controlled Trial." *Psychological Medicine* 47 (2017): 810–821. doi: 10.1017/S0033291716002798.

Fox, Kathryn R., Alexander J. Millner, and Joseph C. Franklin. "Classifying Nonsuicidal Overdoses: Nonsuicidal Self-Injury, Suicide Attempts, or Neither?" *Psychiatry Research* 244 (2016): 235–242. doi: 10.1016/j.psychres.2016.07.052.

Fox, Kathryn R., Jessica D. Ribeiro, Evan M. Kleiman, Jill M. Hooley, Matthew K. Nock, and Joseph C. Franklin. "Affect Toward the Self and Self-Injury Stimuli as Potential Risk Factors for Nonsuicidal Self-Injury." *Psychiatry Research* 260 (2018): 279–285. doi: 10.1016/j.psychres.2017.11.083.

Franklin, Joseph, Megan E. Puzia, Kent M. Lee, and Mitchell J. Prinstein. "Low Implicit and Explicit Aversion Toward Self-Cutting Stimuli Longitudinally Predict Nonsuicidal Self-Injury." *Journal of Abnormal Psychology* 13 (2014): 463–469. Available: http://europepmc.org/abstract/MED/24886018

Franklin, Joseph C., Kathryn R. Fox, Christopher R. Franklin, Evan M. Kleiman, Jessica D. Ribeiro, Adam C. Jaroszewski, Jill M. Hooley, and Matthew K. Nock. "A Brief Mobile App Reduces Nonsuicidal and Suicidal Self-Injury: Evidence from Three Randomized Controlled Trials." *Journal of Consulting Clinical Psychology* 84 (2016): 544–557. doi: 10.1037/ccp0000093.

Glassman, Lisa H., Mariann R. Weierich, Jill M. Hooley, Tara L. Deliberto, and Matthew K. Nock. "Child Maltreatment, Non-Suicidal Self-Injury, and the Mediating Role of Self-Criticism." *Behaviour Research and Therapy* 45 (2007): 2483–2490. doi: 10.1016/j.brat.2007.04.002.

Glenn, Catherine R., Joseph C. Franklin, and Matthew K. Nock. "Evidence-Based Psychosocial Treatments for Self-Injurious Thoughts and Behaviors in Youth." *Journal of Clinical Child & Adolescent Psychology* 44 (2015): 1–29. doi: 10.14440/jbm.2015.54.

Gonzales, Ariel Henrie, and Linda Bergstrom. "Adolescent Non-Suicidal Self-Injury (NSSI) Interventions." *Journal of Child and Adolescent Psychiatric Nursing* 26 (2013): 124–130. doi: 10.1111/jcap.12035.

Hamza, Chloe A., Shannon L. Stewart, and TeenaWilloughby. "Examining the Link Between Nonsuicidal Self-Injury and Suicidal Behavior: A Review of the Literature and an Integrated Model." *Clinical Psychology Review* 32 (2012): 482–495. doi: 10.1016/j.cpr.2012.05.003.

Hofmann, Wilhelm, Jan De Houwer, Marco Perugini, Frank Baeyens, and Geert Crombez. "Evaluative Conditioning in Humans: A Meta-Analysis." *Psychological Bulletin* 136 (2010): 390–421. doi: 10.1037/a0018916.

Hooley, Jill M., Doreen T. Ho, Joshua Slater, and Amanda Lockshin. "Pain Perception and Nonsuicidal Self-Injury: A Laboratory Investigation." *Personality Disorders: Theory, Research, and Treatment* 1 (2010): 170–179. doi: 10.1037/a0020106.

Hooley, Jill M., and Joseph C. Franklin. "Why Do People Hurt Themselves? A New Conceptual Model of Nonsuicidal Self-Injury." *Clinical Psychological Science* 6 (2018): 428–451. doi: 10.1177/2167702617745641.

Hooley, Jill M., and Sarah A. St. Germain. "Nonsuicidal Self-Injury, Pain, and Self-Criticism: Does Changing Self-Worth Change Pain Endurance in People Who Engage in Self-Injury?" *Clinical Psychological Science* 2 (2014): 297–305. doi: 10.1177/2167702613509372.

Kuznetsova, Alexandra, Per Bruun Brockhoff, and Rune Haubo Bojesen Christensen. "lmerTest: Tests for Random and Fixed Effects for Linear Mixed Effect Models (lmer objects of lme4 package)." *R Package Version* 2.0–30 (2012). Available: http://CRAN.R-project.org/package=lmerTest

Lenth, Russell, and M. Hervé. "lsmeans: Least-Squares Means." *R Package Version* 2.16 (2015). doi: 10.18637/jss.v069.i01.

Magnusson, A., H. J. Skaug, A. Nielsen, C. W. Berg, K. Kristensen, M. Maechler, K. van Bentham, B. Bolker, and M. Brooks. "Generalized Linear Mixed Models Using Template Model Builder." *R Package Version* 0.1.3 (2017). Available: https://github.com/glmmTMB

Muehlenkamp, Jennifer J., and Amy M. Brausch. "Body Image as a Mediator of Non-Suicidal Self-Injury in Adolescents." *Journal of Adolescence* 35 (2012): 1–9. doi: 10.1016/j.adolescence.2011.06.010.

Nock, Matthew K. "Self-Injury." *Annual Review Clinical Psychology* 6 (2010): 339–363. doi: 10.1146/annurev.clinpsy.121208.131258.

Nock, Matthew K., Elizabe B. Holmberg, V. I. Photos, and B. D. Michel. "Self-Injurious Thoughts and Behaviors Interview: Development, Reliability, and Validity in an Adolescent Sample." *Psychological Assessment* 19 (2007): 309–317.

Nock, Matthew K., Mitchell J. Prinstein, and Sonya K. Sterba. "Revealing the Form and Function of Self-Injurious Thoughts and Behaviors: A Real-Time Ecological

Assessment Study Among Adolescents and Young Adults." *Journal of Abnormal Psycholoyg* 118, no. 4 (2010): 816–827. doi: 10.1037/2152-0828.1.S.36.

Pennebaker, James W., and Sandra K. Beall. "Confronting a Traumatic Event: Toward an Understanding of Inhibition and Disease." *Journal of Abnormal Psychology* 95 (1986): 274–281. doi: 10.1037/0021-843X.95.3.274.

Ribeiro, J. D., J. C. Franklin, K. R. Fox, K. H. Bentley, E. M. Kleiman, B. P. Chang, and M. K. Nock. "Self-Injurious Thoughts and Behaviors as Risk Factors for Future Suicide Ideation, Attempts, and Death: A Meta-Analysis of Longitudinal Studies." *Psychological Medicine* 46 (2016): 225–236. doi: 10.1017/S0033291715001804.

Selby, Edward A., Theodore W. Bender, Kathryn H. Gordon, Matthew K. Nock, and Thomas E. Joiner. "Non-Suicidal Self-Injury (NSSI) Disorder: A Preliminary Study." *Personal Disorders: Theory, Research and Treatment* 3 (2012): 167–175. doi: 10.1037/a0024405.

Smyth, J. M. "Written Emotional Expression: Effect Sizes, Outcome Types, and Moderating Variables." *Journal of Consulting and Clinical Psychology* 66 (1998): 174–184. doi: 10.1037/0022-006X.66.1.174.

Sowislo, J. F., and U. Orth. "Does Low Self-Esteem Predict Depression and Anxiety? A Meta-Analysis of Longitudinal Studies." *Psychological Bulletin* 139 (2013): 213–240. doi: 10.1037/a0028931.

St. Germain, Sarah A., and Jill M. Hooley. "Direct and Indirect Forms of Non-Suicidal Self-Injury: Evidence for a Distinction." *Psychiatry Research* 197 (2012): 78–84. doi: 10.1016/j.psychres.2011.12.050.

Steer, Robert A., Roberta Ball, William F. Ranieri, and Aaron T. Beck. "Dimensions of the Beck Depression Inventory-II in Clinically Depressed Outpatients." *Journal of Clinical Psychology* 55 (1999): 117–128. doi: 10.1002/(SICI)1097-4679(199901)55:1<117::AID-JCLP12>3.0.CO;2-A.

Swannell, Sarah V., Graham E. Martin, Andrew Page, Penelope Hasking, and Nathan J. St John. "Prevalence of Nonsuicidal Self-Injury in Nonclinical Samples: Systematic Review, Meta-Analysis and Meta-Regression." *Suicide and Life-Threatening Behavior* 44 (2014): 273–303. doi: 10.1111/sltb.12070.

Victor, Sarah Elizabeth, and E. David Klonsky. "Daily Emotion in Non-Suicidal Self-Injury." *Journal of Clinical Psychology* 70 (2014): 364–375. doi: 10.1002/jclp.22037.

Washburn, Jason J., Sarah L. Richardt, Denise M. Styer, Michelle Gebhardt, K. R. Juzwin, Adrienne Yourek, and Delia Aldridge. "Psychotherapeutic Approaches to Non-Suicidal Self-Injury in Adolescents." *Child and Adolescent Psychiatry and Mental Health* 6 (2012): 1–8. doi: 10.1186/1753-2000-6-14.

Chapter 4

Sibling Relationships of Female Adolescents with Non-Suicidal Self-Injury Disorder in Comparison to a Clinical and a Nonclinical Control Group

Taru Tschan, Janine Lüdtke,
Marc Schmid, and Tina In-Albon

INTRODUCTION

Non-suicidal self-injury (NSSI) is a highly prevalent behavior among adolescents and associated with various mental health problems and suicidality (Hamza and Willoughby 2016; In-Albon et al. 2013; Wilkinson et al. 2018). NSSI is defined as the repetitive, deliberate, direct, and socially unaccepted destruction or alteration of one's own body tissue without the intent to die (American Psychiatric Association 2013). Pooled international lifetime prevalence rates among adolescents (including single acts of NSSI) are around 17 percent (Swannell et al. 2014), with 6.7 percent (Zetterqvist 2013) reporting repetitive NSSI according to *DSM-5* criteria (American Psychiatric Association 2013). Females are more likely to report a history of NSSI than men, particularly in clinical samples (Bresin and Schoenleber 2015).

Previous research has emphasized the role of maladaptive family functioning, such as emotional invalidation and lack of family support, as crucial proximal risk factors for the development of NSSI (Baetens et al. 2015; Brausch and Gutierrez 2010; Cassels 2018; Tatnell et al. 2014; Tschan et al. 2015; You and Leung 2012). Contrary, family support and positive family functioning were found to predict the cessation of NSSI (Cassels 2018; Tatnell 2014; Kelada 2016). Similarly, a review on psychosocial treatment for self-injurious thoughts and behaviors concluded that a crucial part of efficacious interventions is improving familial relationships (Glenn et al. 2015). However, research on familial relationships in the context of adolescent NSSI has so far focused primarily on parent–child relationships, while remarkably little is known about sibling relationship quality. The sibling relationship is life's longest lasting and one of the most important relationships, as children spend more time with their siblings than with their parents (Buist et al. 2013). Sibling relationships encompass positive (e.g., warmth, intimacy, empathy) and negative (e.g., conflict, rivalry) features and can have a major impact on siblings' lives and wellbeing (see Dirks et al. 2015 for a review). Social or observational learning are mechanisms to describe generalization of negative behaviors among siblings, such as hostile behavior (Stauffacher and DeHart 2006).

A meta-analysis found that sibling warmth was significantly associated with less internalizing and externalizing problem behavior in children and adolescents (Buist et al. 2013). Within positive sibling relationships, children and adolescents may learn favorable strategies to manage and regulate their emotions, leading to a lower risk of developing symptoms of depression, anxiety, and aggression. On the contrary, sibling conflict was significantly related to more internalizing and externalizing problems (ibid.). Frequent fighting among siblings or observing a siblings hostile behavior might lead to generalization of negative behaviors to other contexts via social learning mechanisms (Stauffacher and DeHart 2006). Noteworthy, the association between internalizing and externalizing problems was stronger for sibling conflict than sibling warmth.

Furthermore, there is some evidence that children and adolescents with mental disorders have poorer sibling relationships compared to nonclinical individuals. Sibling relationships of children with attention deficit hyperactivity disorder (ADHD) are characterized by higher conflict but equal levels of warmth compared to children without ADHD (Mikami and Pfiffner 2008). Noteworthy, the authors suggest that comorbid internalizing and externalizing symptoms might be more powerful predictors of sibling warmth and conflict than ADHD per se. Moreover, poor sibling relationships in childhood and adolescence were found to predict the occurrence of major depression thirty years later (Waldinger et al. 2007). Surprisingly, most research on sibling relationship quality and psychopathology include low-risk community samples (Buist et al. 2013) while there is a lack of research on sibling relationships of children and adolescents with clinically significant mental health issues including NSSI (Dirks et al. 2015).

Adolescent NSSI behavior appears to impact the whole family system, leading to difficulties in parent-child relationships and disrupting family communication, family dynamics, and family functioning (Byrne et al. 2008; Ferrey 2016). Interview studies of parents' reactions to their children's NSSI behavior suggest that parents commonly have feelings of distress, insecurity, anxiety, guilt, and helplessness (ibid.). Because parental time, energy, and attention is focused on the child with self-injuring behavior, parents express worries about an imbalance in parental involvement between siblings, particularly neglecting their other children (Ferrey 2016; McDonald et al. 2007; Oldershaw et al. 2008; Rissanen et al. 2008). Adolescents' NSSI behavior and the distress it causes in the family likely affect siblings, especially if they are of a similar age, as these siblings, too, are trying to navigate through adolescence or young adulthood (Ferrey 2016). According to parents, siblings' reactions to the NSSI behavior include a wide range of feelings such as anger, resentment, frustration, stress, simultaneous empathy and irritation, responsibility, worries about stigma at school, and often, help and support (ibid.). Furthermore, some siblings have indicated feeling anxious about triggering an episode of self-injury with their own behavior (ibid.). To date, studies reporting data on siblings of adolescents with NSSI rely on parental reports, while no studies exist that assess sibling self-report with respect to their reactions to NSSI or sibling relationship quality.

It has been well documented that interpersonal conflicts often serve as triggers for engaging in NSSI (Tschan et al. 2015; Muehlenkamp 2013). Adolescents with NSSI frequently report negative peer experiences, such as peer victimization, which can significantly increase the risk of future NSSI (Giletta 2015). Notably, the source of victimization may also be in the family; a longitudinal study (Bowes et al. 2014) suggested that sibling bullying in early adolescence is significantly associated with NSSI behavior at age eighteen. Identifying risk factors for NSSI within the family might help researchers and clinicians better understand the familial mechanisms that are involved in NSSI and enable them to develop treatment modalities that include the improvement of familial relationships to save and improve the mental health of all family members.

The aim of the current study was threefold. First, we aimed to shed light on how siblings of female adolescents with NSSI feel about and evaluate their sister's NSSI. Second, we wanted to investigate sibling relationship quality rated separately by adolescents with NSSI and a sibling. Previous research has indicated discrepant perspectives on family functioning and parenting behavior between adolescents with NSSI and their parents, with adolescents reporting poorer outcomes than parents (Tschan et al. 2015; Kelada et al. 2016; Palmer et al. 2016). Thus, we further aimed to examine the concordance between adolescent and sibling self-reported sibling relationship quality. Third, we wanted to explore the association between sibling relationship quality and psychopathology for adolescents with NSSI and their siblings, respectively. Specifically, we aimed to answer the following questions:

1. How do siblings react to their sister's NSSI?
2. Do adolescents with NSSI differ from adolescents without NSSI (clinical and nonclinical controls) and from their siblings with respect to sibling relationship quality?
3. To what extent do adolescents and their siblings agree in their reports of relationship quality?
4. Is the sibling relationship quality associated with psychopathology in the NSSI/CC group?

METHODS

Participants

Adolescents

The study included 139 female adolescents, aged thirteen to twenty years ($M = 16.18$ years, $SD = 1.62$) that were consecutively recruited from different inpatient child and adolescent psychiatric units and schools in Switzerland and Germany. The sample comprised of fifty-six adolescents with NSSI disorder, thirty-three adolescents with other mental disorders without NSSI (clinical controls, CC), and fifty adolescents without current or past experience of mental disorders (nonclinical controls, NC). Participants were similar with respect to age, Welch's $F(2, 74.24) = 0.52$. The most frequent mental disorders according to *DSM-IV-TR* of the NSSI group were depressive disorders (76%), anxiety disorders (48.2%), disruptive behavior disorders (22.2%), borderline personality disorder (18.5%), and eating disorders (18.5%). The CC group most frequently reported anxiety disorders (51.5%) and depressive disorders (45.4%), followed by eating disorders (24.2%) and disruptive behavior disorders (12.1%).

Siblings

Seventy-three siblings aged ten to twenty-eight years ($M = 16.88$ years, $SD = 4.02$; 60.3% female) participated in the study. We included only one sibling per adolescent, mainly the one closest in age. Overall, twenty-seven brothers participated (NSSI = 12, CC = 1, NC = 14). Groups of siblings (NSSI = 21, CC = 11, and NC = 41) were similar with respect to age, Welch's $F(2, 20.79) = 0.72$. A minority of siblings in the NSSI group (14.3%; 2 sisters, 1 brother) had had their own experiences with NSSI.

Measures

To examine the adolescents' current or past *DSM-IV-TR* diagnoses for Axis I disorders, we conducted a clinical structured interview. The Diagnostic Interview for Mental Disorders in Children and Adolescents (Kinder-DIPS) (Schneider et al. 2009) assesses the most frequent mental disorders in childhood and adolescence. Questions for substance use disorders were included from the adult DIPS (Schneider and Margraf 2011). The Kinder-DIPS has good validity and reliability for Axis I disorders (child version, $\kappa = 0.48$–0.88) (Neuschwander et al. 2013). NSSI disorder was assessed according to the *DSM-5* research criteria, with questions reformulated as criteria. Interrater reliability estimates for the diagnosis of NSSI were very good ($\kappa = 0.90$). Before conducting the interviews, all interviewers received an intensive standardized training.

Adolescents were administered the Structured Clinical Interview for *DSM-IV* Axis II disorders (SCID-II) (Fydrich et al. 1997) to assess for personality disorders. The SCID-II has been found to be suitable for use among adolescents (Salbach-Andrae et al. 2008). Interrater reliability for borderline personality disorder in our sample was very good ($\kappa = 1.00$).

The Youth Self-Report (YSR) (Achenbach 1991; Döpfner et al. 1994) was used to assess a broad range of psychopathology. Two second-order scales reflecting internalizing and externalizing problems and a total problem score can be calculated. Internal consistency in the present sample was $\alpha = 0.96$ for the total score, $\alpha = 0.85$ for the internalizing score, and $\alpha = 0.80$ for the externalizing score.

The Sibling Questionnaire is a self-developed questionnaire, designed for siblings of adolescents with NSSI and consisting of 166 items (In-Albon and Schmid 2011). Questions with good face validity were gathered and reviewed by experts. The first part contains demographic questions and asks when siblings first noticed their sister's NSSI, and if they were told about it, who told them. Further questions refer to the siblings' suspicions about the reasons for their sister's self-injury ($\alpha = 0.84$), questions about the functions of NSSI were formulated on the basis of the Functional Assessment of Self-Mutilation (Lloyd-Richardson et al. 2007) and the Modified Ottawa/Ulm Self-Injury inventory (Nixon et al. 2002). The second part assesses the siblings' own experiences with NSSI. In the third part, siblings are asked about their feelings ($\alpha = 0.76$) and reactions ($\alpha = 0.63$) when their sister engages in NSSI. The fourth part assesses the impact of NSSI on family dynamics ($\alpha = 0.82$). Reasons for NSSI, siblings' reactions and the impact of NSSI on family dynamics were assessed on a scale ranging from 1 (*fully applies*) to 5 (*does not apply at all*). For siblings' feelings, response choices ranged from

1 (*never*) to 5 (*almost always*). Internal consistencies refer to the present sample. So far, the questionnaire has not been further validated.

The Adult Sibling Relationship Questionnaire (ASRQ) (Heyeres 2006) measures qualitative features of the sibling relationship in young adulthood and consists of eighty-one items spread over fourteen subscales. The three higher order factors are warmth/closeness, conflict, and rivalry. The warmth subscale consists of items measuring affection, companionship, intimacy, and admiration, and the conflict subscale includes quarreling and antagonism between siblings. The rivalry subscale determines whether the parents favor a child, but not which child is favored. All items except rivalry are assessed on a five-point Likert scale ranging from 1 (*hardly at all*) to 5 (*extremely much*). For the rivalry subscale, response choices are 0 (*neither of us is favored*), 1 (*I am/my sibling is sometimes favored*), and 2 (*I am/my sibling is usually favored*). The questionnaire showed good internal consistency (ibid). In the present sample, internal consistency was $\alpha = 0.93$ for warmth, $\alpha = 0.83$ for conflict, and $\alpha = 0.83$ for rivalry.

The Brother-Sister Questionnaire (BSQ) (Graham-Bermann and Cutler 1994) consists of thirty-five items and is used to distinguish dysfunctional from well-functioning sibling relationships. The BSQ measures four dimensions: empathy (emotional connectedness, caring), boundary maintenance (respect for siblings' physical and psychological space), similarity (common interests and experiences), and coercion (power and control of one sibling over another). The questionnaire demonstrated good psychometric properties (ibid.). Internal consistency in the present sample was $\alpha = 0.95$ for empathy, $\alpha = 0.83$ for boundary maintenance, $\alpha = 0.68$ for similarity, and $\alpha = 0.52$ for coercion.

Procedure

Participants from the NSSI and CC sample were recruited from nine collaborating child and adolescent psychiatric inpatient clinics. The inpatient clinics were instructed to inform the participants at admission about the study and asked for their consent to participate. Participants from the NC sample were recruited in different high schools. Prior to our visit in the schools, teachers were given detailed information about the study and handed out written informed consent forms, to be signed by the parents of the students participating. After obtaining written informed consent from the adolescents and caregivers, clinical interviews and self-report questionnaires were performed in the inpatient clinics for the NSSI and CC sample and in a classroom after school for the NC group. After data collection for the participants was completed, they were given consent forms and questionnaires for their siblings in case they were willing to participate in the study. Consent form and questionnaires from the siblings were then returned via mail. All participants, adolescents, their siblings and parents were informed about the study and gave their written consent in accordance with the Declaration of Helsinki. The local ethics committee approved the study.

Data Analyses

We used multivariate analysis of variance (MANOVA) to investigate group differences in sibling relationship. Post-hoc tests were conducted to analyze pairwise comparisons. The Bonferroni correction was used to control for multiple comparisons. Effect sizes (Cohen's d) were calculated to further analyze significant group differences. Pearson product-moment correlation coefficients were calculated to evaluate sibling agreement and associations between sibling relationship quality and psychopathology. To compare correlations of sibling agreement, the coefficients were converted to z scores. In order to examine adolescent-sibling discrepancies, raw and standardized difference scores were calculated. The standardized difference scores were calculated by subtracting the siblings' standardized score from the youth's standardized score (De Los Reyes and Kazdin 2004). The magnitude of discrepancy between standardized scores was examined by calculating the mean of the absolute value of the difference between standardized scores. All analyses were performed using SPSS version 25. Significance levels were set at $\alpha = 0.05$.

RESULTS

Siblings' Reactions to Their Sister's NSSI

Siblings suspected the following reasons for their sister's self-injury: to change the emotional pain into something physical (60.0%), to relieve tension (57.1%), to deal with frustration (45.0%), and to cope with uncomfortable memories (42.9%). About half of the siblings (57.1%) noticed their sister's NSSI, and the majority (90.5%) were concerned about the behavior. A large proportion (85.7%) believed that their sister might attempt suicide and reported being relieved that their sister was hospitalized. The most common emotional reactions to NSSI were feeling sad (76.2%), depressed (66.7%), desperate (57.1%), helpless (57.1%), angry (33.4%), scared (19.1%), and guilty (14.3%). Several siblings endorsed that they sympathized with their sister (61.9%) and felt distressed due to NSSI (42.9%).

From the perspective of many siblings, the sister's issues determined the whole family life (42.9%) and they perceived the family situation as very distressing (42.9%). Around a quarter thought that their parents had found a good way to handle their sister's NSSI (28.6%). Another quarter (23.8%)

reported that they did not get their parents' attention as often as their sisters did and shared the opinion that their parents did not dare to put limits on their sister (23.8%). A third (33.3%) reported supporting their sister by talking with them about NSSI. However, they perceived the conversations as helpful for their sister (28.6%), but stressful for themselves, and indicated that they would like to get help to better cope with their sister's NSSI (28.6%). Many siblings endorsed that they would never understand why their sister is engaging in NSSI (38.1%), and a sizeable proportion felt left alone with the sister's issues (71.4%). Less than half of the siblings (38.1%) reported being reasonably involved in their sister's therapy. Those siblings without their own NSSI experience (85.7%) provided several reasons why they did not engage in NSSI (see table 4.1). Siblings reported having fewer friends who engage in NSSI (14.3%) than their sister reported for herself (47.6%). Siblings of adolescents with NSSI who also engaged in NSSI (14.3%) were all older siblings who indicated that they had started self-injuring earlier than their sister.

Sibling Relationship Quality

Group Comparisons based on Reports of Adolescents with NSSI

Results of the MANOVA showed a significant group difference for the ASRQ subscales warmth, $F(2, 134) = 7.42$, $p < .01$, and rivalry, $F(2, 134) = 14.27$, $p < .01$. Bonferroni-corrected post hoc analysis revealed that adolescents with NSSI reported significantly less warmth ($p < .01$, $d = 0.73$) and more rivalry ($p < .01$, $d = 1.05$) in the sibling relationship than NC adolescents. The higher rivalry score indicates parental favoritism for one child by parents of adolescents with NSSI. No difference between groups (NSSI, CC, NC) was found for the ASRQ subscale conflict (see table 4.2). Regarding the BSQ subscales,

Table 4.1 Siblings of Adolescents with NSSI and Their Reasons for Why They Not Engage in Self-Injurious Behavior (*n* = 18)

Reason	Number of siblings	%
I have better strategies to deal with stress	9	42.9
I have learned to be thick skinned	9	42.9
I feel less burdened by the family situation	8	38.1
I can express and vent my anger	8	38.1
I have better peer relationships	7	33.4
My sister has experienced more bad things	6	28.6
My sister is too sensitive	5	23.8
I am better at solving problems with our parents	5	23.8
My sister feels more burdened by conflicts with our parents	5	23.8

Source: Author created.

the three groups differed significantly on the subscales empathy, similarity, and boundary maintenance. Post-hoc analysis showed that adolescents with NSSI reported significantly less empathy ($p < .01$, $d = 0.68$) and similarity ($p < .01$, $d = 0.78$) than NC adolescents. Adolescents with NSSI reached higher scores in boundary maintenance than NC adolescents ($p < .05$, $d = 0.43$); higher scores reflect less concern with boundary maintenance. As shown in table 4.2, no group difference emerged for the subscale coercion.

Group Comparisons based on Siblings' Reports

The only significant difference emerged on the BSQ subscale coercion, $F(2, 65) = 4.43$, $p = .016$, $\eta^2 = 0.12$, with post hoc analysis showing that siblings of adolescents with NSSI reported significantly more coercion than CC siblings ($p < .05$, $d = 1.08$) and NC siblings ($p < .05$, $d = 0.67$); see table 4.2. No significant differences were found for the remaining BSQ subscales or any ASRQ subscale.

Comparisons between Adolescents and Siblings in the NSSI Group

Significant differences in reports on relationship quality of adolescents with NSSI and their siblings emerged for similarity, $F(1, 68) = 6.3$, $p < .05$, $\eta^2 = 0.09$, and boundary maintenance, $F(1, 68) = 81.07$, $p < .01$, $\eta^2 = 0.54$, with adolescents with NSSI reporting lower scores on the similarity scale and higher scores on the boundary maintenance scale, indicating less concern with boundary maintenance than their siblings.

Sibling Agreement

The results of sibling agreement are displayed in table 4.3. The level of sibling agreement in the NSSI and NC group was low, $r = .05$ to $.35$. Siblings of the CC group showed a significant agreement regarding warmth ($r = .74$) and similarity ($r = .82$). The agreement for both subscales was significantly higher among siblings of the CC group than among NSSI and NC siblings; see table 4.3.

In addition to sibling agreement, table 4.4 reflects sibling discrepancies showing raw and standardized difference scores as well as absolute value standardized differences. There was considerable variability among the difference scores, as indicated by large standard deviations of the raw discrepancy. The mean of the absolute value of the difference between standard scores indicates that the difference between adolescent and sibling reports in the CC and NC group was small for most aspects of relationship quality with less than one standard deviation (< 1). The NSSI group showed the largest discrepancies (> 1 for most subscales).

Table 4.2 Means (and Standard Deviations) Derived from the ASRQ and BSQ on Sibling Relationship Quality and the YSR on Psychopathological Symptoms

Measure	Adolescents					Siblings				
	NSSI (n = 56) M (SD)	CC (n = 33) M (SD)	NC (n = 50) M (SD)	F(2, 134)	η^2	NSSI (n = 21) M (SD)	CC (n = 11) M (SD)	NC (n = 41) M (SD)	F(2, 65)	η^2
ASRQ										
Warmth	141.27 (38.12)	152.75 (26.82)	164.97 (25.69)	7.42**	0.10	155.62 (21.72)	159.15 (31.88)	154.00 (28.50)	0.14	0.00
Conflict	57.81 (14.49)	57.88 (14.46)	56.64 (13.20)	0.12	0.00	56.11 (13.36)	51.78 (9.51)	55.28 (14.20)	0.33	0.01
Rivalry	0.53 (0.47)	0.38 (0.41)	0.14 (0.23)	14.27**	0.18	0.26 (0.47)	0.10 (0.20)	0.31 (0.44)	0.91	0.03
BSQ										
Empathy	3.12 (0.99)	3.39 (0.88)	3.70 (0.70)	5.39**	0.08	3.36 (0.56)	3.44 (0.70)	3.36 (0.67)	0.06	0.00
Boundaries	4.23 (0.71)	4.20 (0.67)	3.89 (0.88)	3.47*	0.05	2.25 (0.86)	1.89 (0.68)	2.06 (0.59)	0.96	0.03
Similarity	2.41 (0.67)	2.55 (0.46)	2.87 (0.50)	9.29**	0.12	2.78 (0.42)	2.57 (0.39)	2.61 (0.57)	0.83	0.03
Coercion	1.95 (0.68)	1.75 (0.68)	1.71 (0.63)	1.11	0.02	2.11 (0.59)	1.57 (0.19)	1.75 (0.52)	4.43*	0.12
YSR										
INT	35.33 (10.14)	21.70 (9.29)	8.95 (5.87)	120.76**	0.64	10.13 (7.49)	9.04 (6.84)	10.53 (7.92)	0.14	0.00
EXT	19.94 (10.54)	11.61 (6.43)	9.33 (5.39)	23.42**	0.26	9.18 (5.03)	7.60 (5.14)	9.18 (5.03)	0.73	0.02

Note. NSSI = Adolescents with non-suicidal self-injury; CC = clinical control group; NC = nonclinical control group; ASRQ = Adult Sibling Relationship; Questionnaire; BSQ = Brother Sister Questionnaire; YSR = Youth Self Report; INT = Internalizing symptoms, EXT = Externalizing symptoms.
*$p < .05$, **$p < .01$.
Source: Author Created.

Table 4.3 Sibling Agreement on Dimensions of Relationship Quality (Pearson Correlations)

Measure	NSSI (n = 42)	CC n = 22 (n = 22)	NC n = 82 (n = 82)	z scores NSSI vs. CC	z scores NSSI vs. NC	z scores CC vs. NC
ASRQ						
Warmth	.07	.74*	.19	−2.07*	−0.43	1.95*
Conflict	.13	.52	.31	−1.05	−0.66	0.66
Rivalry	.11	−.03	.08	0.33	0.11	−0.28
BSQ						
Empathy	.12	.42	.31	−0.77	−0.70	0.33
Boundaries	.20	.58	.06	−1.08	0.50	1.55
Similarity	.35	.82*	.25	−1.86*	0.39	2.32*
Coercion	.05	.29	−.24	−0.56	1.03	1.40

Note. NSSI = Adolescents with non-suicidal self-injury; CC = clinical control group; NC = nonclinical control group.
ASRQ = Adult Sibling Relationship Questionnaire; BSQ = Brother-Sister Questionnaire.
*$p < .05$. **$p < .01$.
Source: Author created.

Association between Sibling Relationship Quality and Psychopathology in the NSSI and CC Group

Correlations between sibling relationship quality and psychopathology are presented separately for adolescents with NSSI and their siblings in tables 4.5 and 4.6. Among adolescents with NSSI, a significant association was found between internalizing problems and coercion as well as externalizing problems and similarity (both $r = .27$). For adolescents in the CC group, significant associations emerged between internalizing problems and conflict ($r = .35$) and boundary maintenance ($r = −.47$) as well as externalizing problems and conflict ($r = .47$), similarity ($r = .37$) and coercion ($r = .35$). In the NSSI group, siblings' reports showed that internalizing problems were significantly associated with warmth, conflict, and empathy (all $r = .48$) in the sibling relationship. No associations between sibling relationship quality and psychopathology were found in reports of siblings in the CC group. Siblings of the three groups did not differ significantly regarding internalizing, $F(2, 65) = 0.14$, $p > .05$, or externalizing, $F(2, 65) = 0.73$, $p > .05$, problems.

DISCUSSION

This study is the first to address siblings' reactions to a sister's NSSI as well as aspects of sibling relationship quality, such as warmth, rivalry, coercion, and conflict, group differences (adolescents with NSSI, CC, NC) with respect to sibling relationship quality, agreement between adolescents with NSSI,

CC, and NC and their siblings, and the association between sibling relationship quality and psychopathology separately for adolescents with NSSI and their siblings.

Consistent with previous research on parental reports of siblings' emotional reactions to NSSI (Byrne et al. 2008; Ferrey 2016), siblings involved in this study described their sister's NSSI as being a source of distress, sadness, desperation, helplessness, and anger. The majority of siblings was concerned about their sister's NSSI as well as potential future suicidal behavior and felt relieved about their sister receiving inpatient psychiatric treatment. A third of siblings supported their sister by talking to her about NSSI and although they considered these conversations helpful for their sister, they perceived them as distressing for themselves and wished for help to cope better with NSSI. In fact, 71.4 percent of siblings felt left alone with the sister's issues and 38.1 percent never understood why their sister was engaging in NSSI. These findings highlight the need to provide sufficient psychoeducation for family members to increase their understanding of the behavior and enhance the family's communication and coping skills (Solomon 1996). Relatives of individuals with a mental disorder have been shown to benefit from psychoeducational support groups (Cuijpers and Stam 2000; Pollio et al. 2006). Based on the siblings' reports in our study, NSSI has a negative impact on emotional well-being and family life, which raises the question of whether these siblings might be at risk of developing their own mental health issues. Research on siblings of individuals with mental disorders has reported high levels of emotional distress, especially if the sibling is still living with the family (Liegghio 2017). However, we found no group differences between siblings in the three groups with respect to internalizing or externalizing symptoms. Nonetheless, given the reported emotional impact of NSSI, the feeling of being left alone with their sister's issues, and the wish for support, it is crucial to create opportunities for siblings to address their worries about NSSI and to receive support. Due to their extensive contact during childhood and adolescence, siblings are often key family members and can be a great source of emotional and practical support (McHale et al. 2012; Tucker et al. 2001). Siblings can help promote the well-being and recovery of a sibling with a mental disorder, through engaging jointly in appropriate activities, for example, exercise or sports, or integrating the sibling in their social circle (Griffiths and Sin 2013).

Adolescents with NSSI reported significantly less warmth, empathy, and similarity and more rivalry in the sibling relationship than NC adolescents. Furthermore, they indicated significantly less concern with boundary maintenance compared to NC adolescents. Adolescents with NSSI felt less emotionally connected with their sibling and reported lower empathy, caring, intimacy, similarity, and companionship in their sibling relationship compared

Table 4.4 Raw, Standardized and Absolute Value Standardized Differences Scores for Adolescent and Sibling Reports of Sibling Relationship Quality

	Raw M (SD)			Difference scores						
				Standardized M (SD)			Absolute value standardized M (SD)			
Measure	NSSI (n = 42)	CC (n = 22)	NC (n = 82)	NSSI (n = 42)	CC (n = 22)	NC (n = 82)	NSSI (n = 42)	CC (n = 22)	NC (n = 82)
ASRQ									
Warmth	3.11 (37.52)	−6.08 (23.15)	9.50 (34.40)	−0.08 (1.36)	−0.41 (0.84)	0.16 (1.24)	1.09 (0.76)	0.74 (0.54)	0.86 (0.90)
Conflict	−1.79 (19.90)	5.20 (11.68)	1.88 (15.68)	−0.28 (1.52)	0.25 (0.89)	−0.00 (1.20)	1.11 (1.04)	0.74 (0.48)	0.92 (0.76)
Rivalry	0.27 (0.48)	0.20 (0.42)	−0.16 (0.49)	0.76 (1.36)	0.51 (1.15)	−0.40 (1.17)	1.15 (0.99)	0.75 (0.97)	0.87 (0.90)
BSQ									
Empathy	0.36 (0.96)	0.12 (0.86)	0.30 (0.81)	0.11 (1.37)	−0.22 (1.25)	0.04 (1.18)	1.11 (0.76)	0.89 (0.85)	0.76 (0.90)
Boundaries	1.88 (1.23)	2.24 (0.73)	1.84 (0.95)	−0.16 (1.70)	0.40 (0.99)	−0.15 (1.28)	1.32 (1.03)	0.81 (0.63)	0.98 (0.83)
Similarity	−0.08 (0.64)	0.07 (0.32)	0.21 (0.64)	−0.27 (1.18)	−0.02 (0.60)	0.26 (1.17)	0.93 (0.76)	0.50 (0.28)	0.91 (0.76)
Coercion	−0.25 (1.05)	0.07 (0.32)	−0.05 (0.83)	−0.38 (1.82)	0.32 (0.54)	0.08 (1.48)	1.37 (1.23)	0.49 (0.36)	1.11 (0.95)

Note. NSSI = Adolescents with non-suicidal self-injury; CC = clinical control group; NC = nonclinical control group. ASRQ = Adult Sibling Relationship Questionnaire; BSQ = Brother-Sister Questionnaire.
Source: Author created.

Table 4.5 Pearson Correlations of Sibling Relationship Quality (ASRQ, BSQ) and Psychopathological Symptoms (YSR) Reported by Adolescents with Non-Suicidal Self-Injury Disorder

Measure	1	2	3	4	5	6	7	8
ASRQ								
1. Warmth	-							
2. Conflict	−.54**	-						
3. Rivalry	−.33*	.15	-					
BSQ								
4. Empathy	.88**	−.61**	−.30*	-				
5. Boundaries	.03	−.36**	−.09	.20	-			
6. Similarity	.62**	−.31*	−.35*	.63**	.16	-		
7. Coercion	−.42**	.50**	.23	−.50**	−.22	−.17	-	
YSR								
8. Internalizing problems	−.03	.11	.13	−.01	.11	−.04	.27*	-
9. Externalizing problems	.11	.02	.22	.19	.15	.27*	.18	.38**

Note. ASRQ = Adult Sibling Relationship Questionnaire; BSQ = Brother-Sister Questionnaire; YSR= Youth Self-Report.
*$p < .05$. **$p < .01$.
Source: Author created.

Table 4.6 Pearson Correlations of Sibling Relationship Quality (ASRQ, BSQ) and Psychopathological Symptoms (YSR) Reported by Siblings of Adolescents with Non-Suicidal Self-Injury Disorder

Measure	1	2	3	4	5	6	7	8
ASRQ								
1. Warmth	–							
2. Conflict	.02	–						
3. Rivalry	−.33	.06	–					
BSQ								
4. Empathy	.72**	.08	−.11	–				
5. Boundaries	−.20	.54*	.20	.19	–			
6. Similarity	.12	.07	−.04	.15	.19	–		
7. Coercion	−.20	.60**	.11	.12	.76**	.01	–	
YSR								
8. Internalizing problems	.48*	.48*	−.01	.48*	.35	−.13	.18	–
9. Externalizing problems	.32	.13	−.29	.28	.02	.33	.02	.37

Note. ASRQ = Adult Sibling Relationship Questionnaire; BSQ = Brother-Sister Questionnaire; YSR= Youth Self-Report.
*$p < .05$. **$p < .01$.
Source: Author created.

to NC adolescents. There is some research indicating that children and adolescents might have similar experiences with siblings and peers in terms of relationship quality (Pike and Atzaba-Poria 2003; Yeh and Lempers 2004; McCoy et al. 1994). A study by Pike and Atzabe-Poria (2003) found that sibling affection predicted greater positivity in their best friendships, while greater sibling hostility was related to lower positivity and greater conflict with friends. Similarly, among children, sibling warmth was positively associated with best friendship quality, whereas sibling conflict was negatively associated with friendship quality (McCoy et al. 1994). A poorer relationship quality with their siblings might be associated with the peer problems of adolescents with NSSI (Muehlenkamp et al. 2013; Adrian 2011). Adolescents with NSSI report significantly less perceived social support from friends and family as well as having fewer people to seek advice from than healthy controls, which supports the notion that they experience difficulties with forming relationships and developing adaptive interpersonal skills (Muehlenkamp et al. 2013). In order to deal with these negative emotional states emerging from stressful peer experiences, NSSI may be used as a coping mechanism (Giletta et al. 2012).

Adolescents with NSSI reported significantly higher rivalry scores than NC adolescents, suggesting that parents of adolescents with NSSI favor one child over another more than NC parents do. The rivalry subscale comprises items assessing maternal and paternal favoritism. This finding can be interpreted in light of research emphasizing that the self-injuring child becomes the center of familial attention, leading to an imbalance in parental involvement between siblings (Ferrey et al. 2016; McDonald et al. 2007; Oldershaw et al. 2008; Rissanen et al. 2008). Similarly, almost a quarter of siblings of adolescents with NSSI represented in this study experienced less parental attention compared to their sister and believed that their parents were having difficulties setting boundaries. Furthermore, a considerable proportion of siblings endorsed the suggestion that the sister's issues determined family life for the whole family (42.9%). However, no group differences on the rivalry subscale between siblings emerged, indicating no group differences with respect to parental favoritism from the sibling's point of view. Differential parental treatment can have a negative impact on family dynamics and sibling relationships and is associated with greater sibling conflict, antagonism, and controlling behaviors (Brody et al. 1992; Furman and Buhrmester 1985; Kowal and Kramer 1997). The parental favoritism reported in families of adolescents with NSSI might contribute to the maladaptive family functioning, which has been found to contribute to maintaining NSSI (Tatnell et al. 2014; Tschan et al. 2015). Adolescents with NSSI have significantly greater success in having their boundaries respected by their siblings compared to NC siblings, which might be linked to our finding that the siblings of adolescents with NSSI reported significantly more coercion than both CC and NC adolescents. As adolescents with NSSI showed more dominance and control over their siblings, it might be easier for them to maintain their boundaries.

Siblings of adolescents with NSSI scored significantly higher on the coercion subscale compared to CC and NC siblings, emphasizing the dominance and control of adolescents with NSSI in their sibling relationship. Studies have shown that high levels of psychological control from a sibling is associated with ill-being, adjustment problems, and anxiety and depressive symptoms in the victimized sibling (Campione-Barr et al. 2014; Conger et al. 1997; Van der Kaap-Deeder et al. 2017). However, coercion was not associated with internalizing and externalizing problems in siblings of adolescents with NSSI. As no clinical cut-off score for the coercion scale exists, it is difficult to determine whether coercion levels in the sibling relationship of adolescents with NSSI are abnormal or not. However, as siblings in the NSSI group scored higher than both CC and NC siblings, this issue requires further elaboration in future studies.

Our results showed that siblings of adolescents with NSSI involved in this study scored significantly lower on the boundary maintenance scale of the BSQ than their sisters, reflecting difficulties in establishing and respecting firm and reasonable interpersonal boundaries between siblings (Graham-Bermann and Cutler 1994). Lower scores indicate that the siblings fail to have their boundaries respected by their sisters with NSSI. Furthermore, adolescents with NSSI scored significantly lower on the similarity subscale than their siblings, indicating that they see themselves as more de-identified and different from their siblings and having less in common compared to their siblings rating. Previous research has shown that NSSI is associated with identity confusion (Claes et al. 2014) and may provide a source of self-identification (Breen et al. 2013). Considering this, it is not surprising that adolescents with NSSI don't identify themselves with their siblings, but see themselves as different.

Overall, sibling agreement in the NSSI group was low, indicating somewhat diverging perceptions of all relationship quality dimensions used in this study. This result differs from an earlier study that found a substantial sibling agreement for the ASRQ subscales warmth, conflict, and rivalry (Stocker et al. 1997). However, the average age of participants (20.60 years) and siblings (23.00 years) was higher than the average age of participants (16.18 years) and siblings (16.88) in this study. Although adolescent and sibling reports in this study differed for most aspects of sibling relationship quality, the magnitude of these discrepancies was quite small, as measured by standardized scores. Adolescents in the CC group showed the best sibling agreement, especially on the subscales warmth and similarity. This result might be explained by differences in the group sizes and should be further examined with larger CC samples.

Dimensions of sibling relationship quality were only moderately associated with psychopathological symptoms among both adolescents with NSSI and their siblings. Among adolescents with NSSI, externalizing problems were significantly associated with similarity in the sibling relationship, whereas internalizing problems were significantly associated with coercion. The first mentioned association can be interpreted in line with previous research showing that high levels of intimacy (as a proxy for similarity) among siblings close in age might increase the affective intensity of their conflicts (Buhrmester and Furman 1990; Recchia et al. 2013), thereby leading to higher levels of aggression. Coercion in sibling relationships can be seen as important learning experience, since siblings influence each other's aversive and aggressive behavior, for example, through reinforcement (Patterson 1982). However, behavioral changes resulting from hostile sibling interactions can cause internalizing symptoms (Compton et al. 2003).

Among siblings of adolescents with NSSI internalizing problems were significantly associated with conflict, warmth, and empathy. The association between conflict and internalizing problems is consistent with previous research showing that greater sibling conflict during childhood and adolescence leads to higher internalizing symptoms (Buist et al. 2013), especially when siblings are close in age (Furman and Buhrmester 1985). The association between high levels of warmth and empathy and internalizing problems may indicate that in close sibling relationships, the sister's mental health issues and NSSI might lead to worries and a negative emotional impact on their sibling, resulting in elevated levels of internalizing symptoms. For adolescent friendships, co-rumination, excessive discussion of interpersonal problems, and negative feelings were found to be associated with high-quality friendships but also with greater internalizing symptoms (Rose et al. 2007). This may also count for close siblings of adolescents with NSSI, who spend much time discussing their sister's problems.

In light of our finding that the relationship between adolescents with NSSI and their siblings is characterized by less warmth, empathy, and similarity and more coercion than in the NC group—and the well-established link between poor sibling relationship quality and emotional and behavioral problems,—sibling interventions (in terms of increasing warmth and reducing conflict) might be beneficial in reducing psychopathological symptoms (for a review, see Dirks et al. 2015). However, promoting more engaged and positive sibling relationships may, in turn, yield the danger of increasing the emotional distress of the sibling, as outlined above. A review on susceptibility to environmental influences highlights that some characteristics such as genetic or temperament factors may leave an individual more resistant or prone to both negative and positive environmental influences (Belsky and Pluess 2009). Thus, some children and adolescents might perceive negative sibling experiences as more distressing than others or might be more likely to benefit from promoting positive sibling interactions (Dirks et al. 2015). Future research is necessary to determine the circumstances in which incorporating treatment components targeting sibling relationships or family dynamics may be beneficial for improving psychological symptoms (ibid.).

Despite the fact that sibling conflicts and aggression can have severe negative consequences for children's and adolescents' well-being, we only have a very limited understanding of evidence-based programs promoting positive sibling relationships. Preliminary evidence for the improvement of sibling relationship quality among school-aged children has been found for interventions targeting children's social skills (for a review, see Tucker and Finkelhor 2017). These interventions either improve social skills in sibling interactions directly via trained professionals or indirectly by focusing on training parents on mediation skills. However, more research is needed with respect to interventions preventing or intervening with sibling conflict and aggression.

The results of the present study should be interpreted in the context of the following limitations. The sample consisted of female adolescents admitted to an inpatient child and adolescent psychiatric unit and, thus, may not generalize to other samples or to male adolescents. The design of the study was cross-sectional. Therefore, the current study cannot explain the direction of effects between an adolescent's NSSI and sibling relationship quality and family dynamics. This should be investigated in future prospective longitudinal studies and on the basis of a larger sample size, including male and female adolescents. Boys who self-injure are a quite understudied population. The literature indicates that boys and girls differ with respect to basic NSSI characteristics such as methods, location, and functions, supporting the idea that interventions should be gender-specific. Given that male-preferred methods of NSSI include hitting and burning, the nature of the behavior might be perceived as aggressive rather than self-injurious, thereby masking the true intention (Whitlock et al. 2011). In light of these differences, it is possible that NSSI performed by boys might elicit a different response from parents and siblings compared to a self-injuring girl; however, future studies on this matter are needed. To date, there is not sufficient data to answer the question whether brothers might have a different coping of their sisters' NSSI than a female sibling. Studies in children and adolescents suggest that gender composition and age difference of sibling pairs have a moderating effect on sibling relationship quality, which in turn, might influence how siblings cope with maladjustment (Buist et al. 2013). Thus, it is possible that a brother copes differently with his sister's NSSI than with a brother's NSSI and vice versa. Further, adolescents with NSSI may perceive their sibling relationship as less warm and supportive due to a negative cognitive bias; this should be addressed in future studies. More research into rivalry is needed in order to understand which child is favored by parents of adolescents with NSSI and to investigate sibling rivalry, since this study only considered parental rivalry. Another, unavoidable limitation was the use of a non-validated questionnaire for the assessment of sibling relationship quality. Nevertheless, we addressed a neglected research question. Strengths of the study were the use of the *DSM-5* diagnostic research criteria for NSSI and the use of a multi-informant approach, including adolescent and sibling reports as well as the inclusion of a clinical and a nonclinical control group.

CONCLUSIONS

Adolescents with NSSI differed significantly with respect to many dimensions of sibling relationship quality compared to the nonclinical controls (NC), but not compared to the clinical controls (CC). We found that the CC group did not differ from adolescents with NSSI nor to the NC group, indicating that differences between the NSSI and the NC group may be attributed to a characteristic of the NSSI group. However, more research is required to explore this relationship in further detail. We found significant differences between all three groups regarding the BSQ subscale coercion, emphasizing the dominance and control of adolescents with NSSI in their sibling relationship compared to both the CC and NC group. Similarly, our results indicate that siblings fail to have their boundaries respected by their sisters with NSSI. Despite the fact that we found differences only between adolescents with NSSI and NC, significant differences between all three groups were found among siblings, indicating a NSSI-specific association. Since this chapter aims to highlight the impact of NSSI on siblings and the siblings' view on sibling relationship quality, we believe that this chapter adds important findings to the literature.

According to the siblings represented in our study, NSSI is associated with poor emotional well-being and family life, as the family attention frequently centers on concerns related to the sister's mental health issues. These results underline the importance of a sibling support component for siblings of adolescents with NSSI to help them cope with the emotional and familial consequences of their sister's NSSI and to prevent and reduce any negative emotional impact in the long term.

DECLARATIONS

Ethics approval and consent to participate: The local ethics committee (Ethikkommission Beider Basel, EKBB) approved the study.

Consent for publication: All participants and parents gave their written consent.

Availability of data and material: The data sets analyzed during the current study are available from the corresponding author on reasonable request.

Competing interests: The authors declare that they have nonfinancial competing interests.

Funding: This study is supported by grant project 100014_135205 awarded to Tina In-Albon in collaboration with Marc Schmid by the Swiss National Science Foundation.

Authors' contributions: TT and JL completed the data analyses and made substantial contributions to the interpretation of the data and the drafting and revision of the manuscript. TI and MS contributed to the ideas, the acquisition and interpretation of the data, and the drafting and revision of the manuscript. All authors read and approved the final manuscript.

Acknowledgments: We thank the participants in this study as well as the research assistants and graduate students on the project at the University of Basel for their assistance in data collection and management. The authors thank the following clinics for recruitment: Zentrum für Kinder- und Jugendpsychiatrie und -psychotherapie Clienia Littenheid AG, Kinder- und Jugendpsychiatrischer Dienst Koenigsfelden, Kinder- und Jugendpsychiatrie Kriens, St. Elisabethen-Krankenhaus Kinder- und Jugendpsychiatrie Loerrach, Kinder- und Jugendpsychiatrie Chur, Universitaere Psychiatrische Kliniken Kinder- und Jugendpsychiatrie Basel, Universitaetsklinik fuer Kinder- und Jugendpsychiatrie Bern, Kinder- und Jugendpsychiatrische Klinik Solothurn, and Klinik Sonnenhof Kinder- und Jugendpsychiatrisches Zentrum Ganterschwil.

REFERENCES

Achenbach, Thomas M. *Manual for the Youth Self-Report and 1991 Profile*. Burlington: University of Vermont Department of Psychiatry, 1991.

Adrian, Molly, Janice Zeman, Cynthia Erdley, Ludmila Lisa, and Leslie Sim. "Emotional Dysregulation and Interpersonal Difficulties as Risk Factors for Nonsuicidal Self-Injury in Adolescent Girls." *Journal of Abnormal Child Psychology* 39 (2011): 389–400.

American Psychiatric Association. *Diagnostic and Statistical Manual of Mental Disorders* (5th ed.). Arlington, VA: American Psychiatric Publishing, 2013.

Baetens, Imke, Tori Andrews, Laurence Claes, and Graham Martin. "The Association Between Family Functioning and NSSI in Adolescence: The Mediating Role of Depressive Symptoms." *Family Science* 6 (2015): 330–7.

Belsky, Jay, and M. Michael Pluess. "Beyond Diathesis Stress: Differential Susceptibility to Environmental Influences." *Psychological Bulletin* 135 (2009): 885–908.
Bowes, Lucy, Dieter Wolke, Carol Joinson, Suzet Tanya Lereya, and Glyn Lewis. "Sibling Bullying and Risk of Depression, Anxiety, and Self-Harm: A Prospective Cohort Study." *Pediatrics* 134 (2014): e1032–9.
Brausch, Amy M., and Peter M. Gutierrez. "Differences in Non-Suicidal Self-Injury and Suicide Attempts in Adolescents." *Journal of Youth and Adolescence* 39 (2010): 233–42.
Breen, Andrea V., Stephen P. Lewis, and Olga Sutherland. "Brief Report: Non-suicidal Self-Injury in the Context of Self and Identity Development." *Journal of Adult Development* 20 (2013): 57–62.
Bresin, Konrad, and Michelle Schoenleber. "Gender Differences in the Prevalence of Nonsuicidal Self-Injury: A Meta-Analysis." *Clinical Psychology Review* 38 (2015): 55–64.
Brody, Gene H., Zolinda Stoneman, and J. Kelly McCoy. "Associations of Maternal and Paternal Direct and Differential Behavior with Sibling Relationships: Contemporaneous and Longitudinal Analyses." *Child Development* 63 (1992): 82–92.
Buhrmester, Duane, and Wyndol Furman. "Perceptions of Sibling Relationships During Middle Childhood and Adolescence." *Child Development* 61 (1990): 1387–98.
Buist, Kirstin L., Maja Deković, and Peter Prinzie. "Sibling Relationship Quality and Psychopathology of Children and Adolescents: A Meta-Analysis." *Clinical Psychology Review* 33 (2013): 97–106.
Byrne, Sinéad, Sophia Morgan, Carol Fitzpatrick, Carole Boylan, Sinéad Crowley, Hilary Gahan, Julie Howley, Dorothy Staunton, and Suzanne Guerin. "Deliberate Self-Harm in Children and Adolescents: A Qualitative Study Exploring the Needs of Parents and Carers." *Clinical Child Psycholology and Psychiatry* 13 (2008): 493–504.
Campione-Barr, Nicole, Anna K. Lindell, Kelly Bassett Greer, and Amanda J. Rose. "Relational Aggression and Psychological Control in the Sibling Relationship: Mediators of the Association Between Maternal Psychological Control and Adolescents' Emotional Adjustment." *Development and Psychopathology* 26 (2014): 749–58.
Cassels, Matthew, Anne-Laura van Harmelen, Sharon Neufeld, Ian Goodyer, Peter B. Jones, and Paul Wilkinson. "Poor Family Functioning Mediates the Link Between Childhood Adversity and Adolescent Nonsuicidal Self-Injury." *Journal of Child Psychology and Psychiatry* 59 (2018): 881–7.
Claes, Laurence, Koen Luyckx, and Patricia Bijttebier. "Non-Suicidal Self-Injury in Adolescents: Prevalence and Associations with Identity Formation Above and Beyond Depression." *Personality and Individual Differences* 61–62 (2014): 101–4.
Compton, Kristi, James Snyder, Lynn Schrepferman, Lew Bank, and Joann Wu Shortt. "The Contribution of Parents and Siblings to Antisocial and Depressive

Behavior in Adolescents: A Double Jeopardy Coercion Model." *Development and Psychopathology* 15 (2003): 163–82.

Conger, Katherine Jewsubry, Rand D. Conger, and Larua V. Scaramella. "Parents, Siblings, Psychological Control, and Adolescent Adjustment." *Journal of Adolescent Research* 12 (1997): 113–38.

Cuijper, Pim, and Heleen Stam. "Burnout Among Relatives of Psychiatric Patients Attending Psychoeducational Support Groups." *Psychiatric Services* 51 (2000): 375–9.

De Los Reyes, Andres, and Alan E. Kazdin. "Measuring Informant Discrepancies in Clinical Child Research." *Psychological Assessment* 16 (2004): 330–4.

Dirks, Melanie A., Ryab Persram, Hollty E. Recchia, and Nina Howe. "Sibling Relationships as Sources of Risk and Resilience in the Development and Maintenance of Internalizing and Externalizing Problems During Childhood and Adolescence." *Clinical Psychology Review* 42 (2015): 145–55.

Döpfner, M., P. Melchers, J. Fegert, G. Lehmkuhl, U. Lehmkuhl, K. Schmeck, H.-Ch. Steinhausen, and F. Poustka. "Deutschsprachige Konsensus-Versionen der Child Behavior Checklist (CBCL 4-18), der Teacher Report Form (TRF) und der Youth Self Report Form (YSR)." *Kindh Entwickl* 3 (1994): 54–9.

Ferrey, Anne E., Nicholas D. Hughes, Sue Simkin, Louise Locock, Anne Stewart, Navneet Kapur, David Gunnell, and Keith Hawton "The Impact of Self-Harm by Young People on Parents and Families: A Qualitative Study." *BMJ* 6 (2016): e009631.

Furman, Wyndol, and Duane Buhrmester. "Children's Perceptions of the Qualities of Sibling Relationships." *Child Development* 56 (1985): 448–61.

Fydrich, T., B. Renneberg, B. Schmitz, H. U. Wittchen. *SKID-II. Strukturiertes Klinisches Interview für DSM-IV, Achse II: Persönlichkeitsstörungen.* Göttingen, Germany: Hogrefe, 1997.

Giletta, Matteo, Mitchell J. Prinstein, John R. Z. Abela, Brandon E. Gibb, Andrea L. Barrocas, and Benjamin L. Hankin. "Trajectories of Suicide Ideation and Nonsuicidal Self-Injury Among Adolescents in Mainland China: Peer Predictors, Joint Development, and Risk for Suicide Attempts." *Journal of Consulting and Clinical Psychology* 83 (2015): 265–79.

Giletta, Matteo, Ron H. J. Scholte, Rutger C. M. E. Engels, Silvia Ciairano, and Mitchell J. Prinstein. "Adolescent Non-Suicidal Self-Injury: A Cross-National Study of Community Samples from Italy, the Netherlands and the United States." *Psychiatry Research* 197, no. 1–2 (2012): 66–72.

Glenn, Catherine R., Joseph C. Franklin, and Matthew K. Nock. "Evidence-Based Psychosocial Treatments for Self-Injurious Thoughts and Behaviors in Youth." *Journal of Clinical Child & Adolescent Psychology* 44 (2015): 1–29.

Graham-Bermann, Sandra A., and Susan E. Cutler. "The Brother-Sister Questionnaire: Psychometric Assessment and Discrimination of Well-Functioning from Dysfunctional Relationships." *Journal of Family Psychology* 8 (1994): 224–38.

Griffiths, C., and J. Sin. "Rethinking Siblings and Mental Illness." *The Psychologist* 26 (2013): 808–10.

Hamza, Chloe A., and Teena Willoughby. "Nonsuicidal Self-Injury and Suicidal Risk Among Emerging Adults." *Journal of Adolescent Health* 59 (2016): 411–5.

Heyeres, Uwe. "Adult Sibling Relationship Questionnaire." Gruppendynamik und Organisationsberatung 37 (2006): 215–25.

In-Albon, Tina, Claudia Ruf, and Marc Schmid. "Proposed Diagnostic Criteria for the *DSM-5* of Nonsuicidal Self-Injury in Female Adolescents: Diagnostic and Clinical Correlates." *Psychiatry Journal* 2013 (2013). doi: 10.1155/2013/159208.

In-Albon, Tina, and Marc Schmid. *The Sibling Questionnaire*. Unpublished manuscript. Basel: University of Basel, 2011.

Kelada, Lauren, Penelope Hasking, and Glenn Melvin. "Adolescent NSSI and Recovery: The Role of Family Functioning and Emotion Regulation." *Youth & Society* 50 (2016a): 1056–77.

Kelada, Lauren, Penelope Hasking, and Glenn Melvin. "The Relationship Between Nonsuicidal Self-Injury and Family Functioning: Adolescent and Parent Perspectives." *Journal of Marital and Family Therapy* 42 (2016b): 536–49.

Liegghio, Maria. "'Not a Good Person': Family Stigma of Mental Illness from the Perspectives of Young Siblings." *Child & Family Social Work* 22 (2017): 1237–45.

Lloyd-Richardson, Elizabeth E., Nicholas Perrine, Lisa Dierker, and Mary L. Kelley. "Characteristics and Functions of Nonsuicidal Self-Injury in a Community Sample of Adolescents." *Psychological Medicine* 37, no. 8 (2007): 1183–92.

McCoy, J. Kelly, Gene H. Brody, and Zolinda Stoneman. "A Longitudinal Analysis of Sibling Relationships as Mediators of the Link between Family Processes and Youths' Best Friendships." *Family Relations* 43 (1994): 400–8.

McDonald, Glenda, Louise O'Brien, and Debra Jackson. "Guilt and Shame: Experiences of Parents of Self-Harming Adolescents." *Journal of Child Health Care* 11 (2007): 298–310.

McHale, Susan M., Kimberly A. Updegraff, and Shawn D. Whiteman. "Sibling Relationships and Influences in Childhood and Adolescence." *Journal of Marriage and Family* 74 (2012): 913–30.

Mikami, Amori Yee, and Linda Pfiffner. "Sibling Relationships Among Children with ADHD." *Journal of Attention Disorder* 11 (2008): 482–92.

Muehlenkamp, Jennifer, Amy Brausch, Katherine Quigley, and Janis Whitlock. "Interpersonal Features and Functions of Nonsuicidal Self-Injury." *Suicide and Life-Threatening Behavior* 43, no. 1 (2013): 67–80.

Neuschwander, Murielle, Tina In-Albon, Carmen Adornetto, Binia Roth, and Silvia Schneider. "Interrater-Reliabilitat des Diagnostischen Interviews bei Psychischen Storungen im Kindes- und Jugendalter (Kinder-DIPS)." Z *Kinder Jugendpsychiatr Psychother* 41 (2013): 319–34.

Nixon, Mary K., Paula F. Cloutier, and Sanjay Aggarwal. "Affect Regulation and Addictive Aspects of Repetitive Self-Injury in Hospitalized Adolescents." *Journal of the American Academy of Child and Adolescent Psychiatry* 41 (2002): 1333–41.

Oldershaw, Anna, Clair Richards, Mima Simic, and Ulrike Schmidt. "Parents' Perspectives on Adolescent Self-Harm: Qualitative Study." *The British Journal of Psychiatry* 193, no. 2 (2008): 140–4.

Palmer, Elizabeth, Patrick Welsh, and Paul Alexander Tiffin. "Perceptions of Family Functioning in Adolescents Who Self-Harm." *Journal of Family Therapy* 38 (2016): 257–73.

Patterson, Gerald Roy. *Coercive Family Process*. Eugene, OR: Castalia, 1982.

Pike, Alison, and Naaama Atzaba-Poria. "Do Sibling and Friend Relationships Share the Same Temperamental Origins? A Twin Study." *Journal of Child Psychology and Psychiatry* 44 (2003): 598–611.

Pollio, David E., Carol S. North, Donna L. Reid, Michelle M. Miletic, and Jennifer R. McClendon. "Living with Severe Mental Illness—What Families and Friends Must Know: Evaluation of a One-Day Psychoeducation Workshop." *Social Work* 51 (2006): 31–8.

Recchia, Holly, Cecilia Wainryb, and Monisha Pasupathi. "'Two for Flinching': Children's and Adolescents' Narrative Accounts of Harming Their Friends and Siblings." *Child Development* 84 (2013): 1459–74.

Rissanen, M.-L., J. P. O. Kylmä, and E. R. Laukkanen. "Parental Conceptions of Self-Mutilation Among Finnish Adolescents." *Journal of Psychiatric Mental Health Nursing* 15 (2008): 212–8.

Rose, Amanda J., Wendy Carlson, and Erika M. Waller. "Prospective Associations of Co-Rumination with Friendship and Emotional Adjustment: Considering the Socioemotional Trade-Offs of Co-Rumination." *Developmental Psychology* 43 (2007): 1019–31.

Salbach-Andrae, Harriet, Klaus Lenz, Nicole Simmendinger, Nora Klinkowski, Ulrike Lehmkuhl, and Ernst Pfeiffer. "Psychiatric Comorbidities among Female Adolescents with Anorexia Nervosa." *Child Psychiatry and Human Devevelopment* 39 (2008): 261–72.

Schneider, S., and J. Margraf. *Diagnostisches Interview bei Psychischen Störungen* (4th ed.). Berlin: Springer, 2011.

Schneider, S., S. Unnewehr, and J. Margraf. *Diagnostisches Interview Psychischer Störungen im Kindes- und Jugendalter (Kinder-DIPS)* (4th ed.). Heidelberg: Springer, 2009.

Solomon, Phyllis. "Moving from Psychoeducation to Family Education for Families of Adults with Serious Mental Illness." *Psychiatric Services* 47 (1996): 1364–70.

Stauffacher, Kristin, and Ganie B. DeHart. "Crossing Social Contexts: Relational Aggression Between Siblings and Friends During Early and Middle Childhood." *Journal of Applied Developmental Psychology* 27 (2006): 228–40.

Stocker, Clare M., Richard P. Lanthier, and Wyndol Furman. "Sibling Relationships in Early Adulthood." *Journal of Family Psychology* 11 (1997): 210.

Swannell, Sarah V., Graham E. Martin, Andrew Page, Penelope Hasking, and Nathan J. St. John. "Prevalence of Nonsuicidal Self-Injury in Nonclinical Samples: Systematic Review, Meta-Analysis and Meta-Regression." *Suicide and Life-Threatening Behavior* 44 (2014): 273–303.

Tatnell, Ruth, Lauren Kelada, Penelope Hasking, and Graham Martin. "Longitudinal Analysis of Adolescent NSSI: The Role of Intrapersonal and Interpersonal Factors." *Journal of Abnormal Child Psychology* 42, no. 6 (2014): 885–96.

Tschan, Taru, Marc Schmid, and Tina In-Albon. "Parenting Behavior in Families of Female Adolescents with Nonsuicidal Self-Injury in Comparison to a Clinical and a Nonclinical Control Group." *Child and Adolescent Psychiatry and Mental Health* 9 (2015): 17.

Tucker, Corinna Jenkins, and David Finkelhor. "The State of Interventions for Sibling Conflict and Aggression: A Systematic Review." *Trauma Violence Abuse* 18 (2017): 396–406.

Tucker, Corinna Jenkins, Susan M. McHale, and Ann C. Crouter. "Conditions of Sibling Support in Adolescence." *Journal of Family Psychology* 15 (2001): 254–71.

Van der Kaap-Deeder, Jolene, Marten Vansteenkiste, Bart Soenens, and Elien Mabbe. "Children's Daily Well-Being: The Role of Mothers,' Teachers,' and Siblings' Autonomy Support and Psychological Control." *Developmental Pscychology* 53 (2017): 237–51.

Waldinger, Robert J., George E. Vaillant, and E. John Orav. "Childhood Sibling Relationships as a Predictor of Major Depression in Adulthood: A 30-Year Prospective Study." *The American Journal of Psychiatry* 164 (2007): 949–54.

Whitlock, Janis, Jennifer Muehlenkamp, Amanda Purington, John Eckenrode, Paul Barreira, and Gina Baral Abrams. "Nonsuicidal Self-Injury in a College Population: General Trends and Sex Differences." *Journal of American College Health* 59 (2011): 691–8.

Wilkinson, Paul O., Tianyou Qiu, Sharon Neufeld, Peter B. Jones, and Ian M. Goodyer. "Sporadic and Recurrent Non-Suicidal Self-Injury before Age 14 and Incident Onset of Psychiatric Disorders by 17 Years: Prospective Cohort Study." *The British Journal of Psychiatry* 212 (2018): 222–6.

Yeh, Hsiu-Chen, and Jacques D. Lempers. "Perceived Sibling Relationships and Adolescent Development." *Journal of Youth and Adolescence* 33 (2004): 133–47.

You, Jianing, and Freedom Leung. "The Role of Depressive Symptoms, Family Invalidation and Behavioral Impulsivity in the Occurrence and Repetition of Non-Suicidal Self-Injury in Chinese Adolescents: A 2-year Follow-Up Study." *Journal of Adolescence* 35 (2012): 389–95.

Zetterqvist, Maria, Lars-Gunnar Lundh, Örjan Dahlström, and Carl Goran Svedin. "Prevalence and Function of Non-Suicidal Self-Injury (NSSI) in a Community Sample of Adolescents, Using Suggested DSM-5 Criteria for a Potential NSSI Disorder." *Journal of Abnormal Child Psychology* 41 (2013): 759–73.

Chapter 5

Using Micro-Longitudinal Methods to Examine Social-Communicative Functions of Self-injury in Everyday Life

Brianna J. Turner and Carolyn E. Helps

WHY DO SOME PEOPLE HURT THEMSELVES?

Non-suicidal self-injury (NSSI) is prevalent—affecting around 3 to 6 percent of adults (Klonsky 2011; Plener et al. 2016) and 16 to 18 percent of youth (Muehlenkamp et al. 2012)—and puzzling. Why would a person choose to deliberately hurt his or her body? The last two decades have witnessed a rapid increase in efforts to answer this question. Our understanding of NSSI has been bolstered by the use of varied methods of inquiry, including individuals' narrative accounts of this behavior, detailed clinical observations and case histories, and sophisticated experimental and longitudinal designs. As a result, we know much more about both distal and proximal contributors to NSSI than we did twenty years ago.

Research has now addressed all three domains of the common "bio-psycho-social" framework that guides much of our psychological and psychiatric research. *Biological* correlates of NSSI include an altered response to stress, atypical pain processing (i.e., analgesia or hyperalgesia), alterations in the serotoninergic and dopaminergic neurotransmitter systems and the genes that influence them, low cholesterol and essential fatty acids, and structural and functional abnormalities in several specific brain regions including the anterior cingulate cortex, amygdala, orbitofrontal cortex, and dorsolateral prefrontal cortex (see Groschwitz and Plener 2012 for a systematic review). Key *psychological* risk factors include a personality profile combining being prone to experiencing negative emotion and acting impulsively as well as general and specific facets of internalizing and/or externalizing psychopathology, such as depression, hopelessness, self-criticism, and difficulties regulating one's emotions and relating to one's body (see Fox et al. 2015 for a meta-analytic review). *Social* vulnerabilities to NSSI include adverse childhood experiences such as trauma, neglect, or family conflict, stressful interpersonal experiences such as rejection, bullying, loss, social isolation, and loneliness, and peer influences including having friends who self-injure and identifying with social groups in which NSSI is more common or accepted or that experience high rates of discrimination (e.g., Bowes et al. 2015; Fox et al. 2017; Muehlenkamp et al. 2015; Young et al. 2014; see also Heilbron et al. 2014 for a recent review).

The recent surge of NSSI research has done much to advance our understanding of why some individuals engage in this perplexing behavior. The research also underscores the fact that NSSI is "overdetermined." This means that, rather than being attributable to a single cause, reason, or trigger, our best evidence suggests that NSSI arises due to multiple interacting factors across biological, psychological, and sociocultural systems (Prinstein 2008; Suyemoto 1998).

It is crucial to always remember that complex interactions among many factors explain more about NSSI than any single factor on its own. It would be difficult for anyone to make use of the information above; however, in the absence of an organizing framework that describes how and why these risk factors relate to one another. Fortunately, NSSI research has not only substantially expanded its empirical base, it has also produced theories that help to understand and guide efforts to reduce NSSI. Many of these theories begin with a focus on one essential feature: NSSI seems to temporarily alleviate unwanted or unpleasant emotions, thoughts, and sensations (Chapman et al. 2006; Gratz 2003; Kleindienst et al. 2008; Klonsky et al. 2014).

When researchers and clinicians ask people why they engage in NSSI, the most common response is that NSSI helps people feel better by reducing distress or tension (Klonsky 2007). Thus, it is not surprising that most biological, psychological, and sociocultural risk factors mentioned above can be linked to a vulnerability to experiencing intense negative emotions and thoughts, difficulties effectively managing these emotions and thoughts, and the negative reinforcement cycle that is created when NSSI terminates or dampens such states (Andover and Morris 2014; Chapman et al. 2006; Linehan 1993). The resulting emotion regulation theories of NSSI offer compelling insight that unifies the literature.

Still, given the overdetermined nature of NSSI, understanding NSSI as an effort to regulate unwanted or aversive internal states likely provides just one piece of the puzzle. Indeed, early clinical descriptions of NSSI proposed multiple models that could account for this behavior (Briere and Gil 1998; Favazza 1989; Suyemoto 1998; Walsh and Rosen 1988) including a social-communicative model. According to the social-communicative model, NSSI can signal distress, increase support, assert boundaries, and influence others (Favazza 1989; Klonsky 2007; Suyemoto 1998), and these functions are also important in understanding why some people hurt themselves. These social-communicative functions are increasingly acknowledged in integrative theories of NSSI (Hooley and Franklin 2018; Nock 2009; Nock and Prinstein 2004), which link intrapersonal (e.g., emotion regulation, cognitive theory) and interpersonal (e.g., communications theory, social learning theory) models of NSSI.

The goals of this chapter are twofold. First, we provide an updated review of the evidence supporting social-communicative models of NSSI. Second, we describe how a set of methods known as "micro-longitudinal designs" are especially well-suited to advancing the field beyond what we currently know, providing direct tests of key tenets of our social-communicative models. We begin by providing a brief review of research examining the social context of NSSI, including interpersonal antecedents that render a person more likely to engage in NSSI and interpersonal consequences that influence the likelihood that the behavior will be repeated. We will focus particular attention on three assumptions that underlie social-communicative models of NSSI. Next, we discuss the utility of micro-longitudinal studies for testing social-communicative models of NSSI and describe five exemplar studies that used these methods to deepen our understanding of social-communicative functions of NSSI. We conclude with recommendations and future directions to advance this field.

UNDERSTANDING SELF-INJURY THROUGH A SOCIAL-COMMUNICATIVE LENS

Early interpersonal models based on in-depth clinical observations, surveys, and interviews with people who self-injure suggested that NSSI can sometimes help people thwart, reduce, or cope with perceived rejection or abandonment by signaling distress and eliciting soothing or closeness with others (Favazza and Rosenthal 1993; Rosen et al. 1990). Based on observations in psychiatric inpatient units where NSSI occurred or intensified in several patients around the same time (sometimes called "contagion"), some clinicians posited that NSSI could also serve to signal shared identities, consolidate group cohesion, and assert boundaries of insider versus outsider group members (Rosen and Walsh 1989; Walsh and Rosen 1985). Unfortunately, these early models were sometimes (mis)interpreted to support potentially stigmatizing notions that NSSI could be considered manipulative, attention-seeking, or a cry for help in the absence of genuine distress.

While the stigmatizing idea that NSSI is enacted *primarily* to influence others has been resoundingly rejected (e.g., Kerr et al. 2010; Klonsky et al. 2014; Nock 2008), the concept that some episodes of NSSI are reinforced by the reactions and responses of others, even when this may not have been the actor's intent, remains at the core of contemporary interpersonal models of NSSI (Nock 2008, 2009). For instance, Nock and Prinstein's four-function model (2004, 2005) delineates two social functions of NSSI: a *social positive reinforcement* function, which occurs when NSSI elicits a desired response from others, such as concern, closeness, or soothing and a *social negative reinforcement* function, which occurs when NSSI elicits relief from unwanted interpersonal demands, such as unpleasant activities or interactions with undesirable companions. Two additional intrapersonal functions of NSSI consist of an *automatic positive reinforcement* function, which occurs when NSSI generates desired emotional or cognitive states such as numbness, calmness, or exhilaration and an *automatic negative reinforcement* function, which occurs when NSSI reduces unwanted emotional or cognitive states such as sadness, anger, or tension. Indeed, survey research shows that about 20 to 50 percent of people report *social negative reinforcement* or *social positive reinforcement* functions for NSSI (Klonsky 2007; Jacobson and Batejan 2014), and some evidence suggests that these functions might be underreported due to associated stigma (Heath et al. 2009).

Nock's (2008) anthropological model of self-injury expands upon the social positive reinforcement and social negative reinforcement functions described in the four-function model. According to the anthropological model, NSSI can result in desirable social consequences by eliciting caretaking behaviors through a signal of distress by warding off aggressors or unwanted social demands by portraying a signal of strength and by increasing affiliation with a desirable social group. Within this model, Nock (2008) also introduces the social signaling hypothesis, which suggests that NSSI is enacted as a means of communicating distress when less intense behaviors, such as verbal communication, have failed. According to this hypothesis, NSSI serves as a high-intensity signal of distress that, while costly, can be more effective at meeting interpersonal needs than other less costly signals.

Like the four-function model, the social signaling hypothesis does not imply that a person who engages in NSSI always does so with a deliberate or explicit intention of influencing others. Rather, it assumes that NSSI sometimes produces desirable interpersonal outcomes, whether these were intended or not. In contrast to early conceptualizations of NSSI as a "manipulative" behavior, this hypothesis views NSSI as an understandable method of communicating genuine distress or meeting other important interpersonal needs when previous attempts have been ineffective.

Similar ideas are captured in the cognitive vulnerability-stress model (Guerry and Prinstein 2010), which suggests that people who engage in NSSI often make highly negative attributions in response to interpersonal stressors, for example, that they are *socially inept,* that they are *broadly disliked* by others, or that their relationships are *failing*. These attributions, understandably, result in intense negative emotion. Because these strong negative feelings are more difficult to regulate than less intense negative emotions, people with this cognitive style are more likely to use maladaptive coping strategies like NSSI to manage intense distress, as these strategies may be more effective for reducing very intense emotions.

In addition, people with this cognitive style may have difficulty using "low cost" communication strategies, like talking through a conflict, to meet their interpersonal needs during times of intense negative emotion and, instead, turn to "high cost" signals like NSSI. A similar cascading effect is seen in Yates' (2004) developmental model, which argues that adverse childhood experiences, especially early maltreatment, impair relational skills—for example, difficulty forming close and trusting relationships and difficulty repairing relationship conflict or injuries—throughout childhood, adolescence and adulthood. These skill deficits, in turn, increase the likelihood that a person uses maladaptive strategies such as NSSI to meet their interpersonal needs.

ASSUMPTIONS AND EVIDENCE FOR SOCIAL-COMMUNICATIVE MODELS

Social-communicative models of NSSI share three fundamental assumptions: that NSSI can help a person meet his or her interpersonal needs; that NSSI can produce desirable changes in a person's social environment that make the behavior more likely to recur; and that other people should be aware of the NSSI in order for the behavior to be considered truly "communication." We describe the evidence supporting or refuting each of these assumptions, as well as gaps in our understanding, below.

Assumption 1: NSSI Helps to Meet Unmet Interpersonal Needs

Social-communicative models propose that NSSI can help an individual meet their interpersonal needs that they are otherwise unable to satisfy. Thus, these models also assume that people who engage in NSSI have difficulty meeting interpersonal needs. Whether these difficulties arise due to insufficient or incompatible responses from the environment, requesting behaviors from the individual, or a combination of these is yet unclear. Consistent with this assumption, however, research shows that individuals who engage in NSSI demonstrate various interpersonal difficulties relative to their peers who do not self-injure.

Individuals who engage in NSSI are more likely to have experienced adverse childhood experiences, such as maltreatment (Serafini et al. 2017), parental absence (Trujillo and Servaty-Seib 2017), and bullying (Claes et al. 2015; Giletta et al. 2012; Keenan et al. 2014). They rate their relationships with friends and parents as more conflicted, more distant, and less supportive (Claes et al. 2010; Di Pierro et al. 2012; Muehlenkamp et al. 2013; Rotolone and Martin 2012; Santangelo et al. 2017; Tatnell et al. 2014). They are less skillful in interpersonal communication and resolving interpersonal problems according to both self-ratings and observer ratings (Nock and Mendes 2008; Jacobson et al. 2015; Kim et al. 2015; Laghi et al. 2016). These interpersonal difficulties have been shown to predict the onset of NSSI (Hankin and Abela 2011; Tatnell et al. 2014; Victor et al. 2019; You et al. 2012), suggesting that interpersonal difficulties may be a precursor that establishes vulnerability to NSSI, rather than solely a consequence of the behavior. Moreover, interpersonal difficulties are associated with stronger endorsement of social-communicative functions of NSSI, such as using NSSI to communicate distress or assert boundaries (Hilt et al. 2008; Turner et al. 2012), while the presence of supportive relationships attenuates the relationship between interpersonal difficulties and NSSI (Christoffersen et al. 2015; Hilt et al. 2008). Early evidence suggests that the relationship between interpersonal stress and NSSI may be stronger in people who have a genetic vulnerability to depression and negative emotion relative to people without this vulnerability (Hankin et al. 2014), but more studies of these gene by environment interactions are needed before firm conclusions can be drawn.

In addition to serving as a risk factor for NSSI, interpersonal stress also seems to serve as a *proximal trigger* for NSSI. Negative interpersonal events such as rejection, separation, and failure are often identified as precipitants to NSSI by people who engage in this behavior (Herpertz 1995). This relationship has also been demonstrated in an observational study of an adolescent inpatient treatment program wherein the frequency of NSSI among patients increased when they were anticipating a staff member leaving the program (an interpersonal loss) relative to periods without an anticipated loss (Rosen et al. 1990).

Together, the body of evidence tells us that people who engage in NSSI tend to struggle to establish and maintain close relationships, compared to people who do not engage in NSSI, supporting the idea that individuals who engage in NSSI may have difficulty meeting interpersonal needs via less intense or costly communicative behaviors (Nock 2008). However, showing differences between people with and without a history of NSSI only gives us part of the picture. It is possible, for instance, that NSSI and interpersonal problems are both explained by a third, unobserved variable, such as depression or anxiety. To establish a social-communicative function of NSSI, we need to know whether NSSI itself produces changes in the interpersonal environment that make this behavior more reinforcing. We turn to the evidence regarding the interpersonal consequences of NSSI with the next assumption.

Assumption 2: NSSI Can Produce Desirable Changes in the Interpersonal Environment

Social-communicative models propose that NSSI can, at least in some instances, change a person's interpersonal environment in a positive way, increasing the likelihood that the behavior will be repeated. Such changes might include increases in closeness or perceived support, decreases in criticism or perceived rejection, and changes in the perceived strength of affiliations with desired and undesired groups. Evidence supporting this assumption is mixed, however, and broadly suggests that while positive interpersonal consequences of NSSI are possible, they may co-occur with negative interpersonal consequences. For instance, compared to adolescent girls who engaged in other risky behaviors (e.g., cigarette, alcohol, or drug use), adolescent girls who engaged in NSSI reported more improvements in father-daughter relationships over one year (Hilt et al. 2008). Similarly, adolescents' NSSI predicted parents' use of positive parenting strategies such as rule setting and monitoring (Baetens et al. 2015); however, adolescents' NSSI also predicted more parental punishment (ibid.) and more interpersonal stressors, even after controlling for depressive symptoms (Burke et al. 2015).

A self-report study also underscores possible negative interpersonal consequences of NSSI. About one fifth of people who engaged in NSSI reported that their relationships suffered as a result of their self-injury or that their social life would be better if they did not self-injure, and about one-third endorsed feeling embarrassed by their self-injury (Burke et al. 2017). Moreover, a prospective study showed that increases in interpersonal stressors predicted worsening depression (Burke et al. 2015), suggesting a possible self-reinforcing pattern whereby NSSI produces more conflict with parents and peers, which then increases the severity of depression, making NSSI more reinforcing. A similar pattern was not found for non-interpersonal stressors, suggesting that more frequent NSSI may uniquely lead to deterioration in relationships, rather than a broader pattern of stress generation. Further complicating matters, another study found no relationship between NSSI and later relationship difficulties (You et al. 2012).

Together, these findings suggest that, in some cases, NSSI leads to closer relationships, while in other cases, NSSI increases relationship stress or has no effect on relationships. Teasing apart the conditions under which NSSI produces desirable versus undesirable interpersonal consequences, ideally using multiple informants (e.g., people who engage in NSSI as well as their partners, peers, and parents) and prospective designs, is an important direction for future research.

Assumption 3: Other People Should be Aware of NSSI Behavior

A third and final assumption of social-communicative models of NSSI is that other people should be aware of the behavior. While it is possible for a behavior to change other people's attitudes and actions without their explicit awareness, it is difficult to say that a behavior functions *to communicate* if no one else knows about it. An important challenge to social-communicative models of NSSI, therefore, is the fact that many people who engage in NSSI often go to considerable lengths to conceal their NSSI (Klineberg et al. 2013; Lewis and Mehrabkhani 2016; Rodham et al. 2016).

How often do people who engage in NSSI actually disclose this behavior? By early adulthood, around 60 to 90 percent of people who engage in NSSI have told at least one other person that they engage in this behavior, most often a friend, romantic partner or parent (Hasking 2015; Muehlenkamp et al. 2013; Whitlock 2006; Wilcox et al. 2012). Only 10 to 15 percent of people disclose NSSI to a mental health professional (Hasking et al. 2015; Muehlenkamp et al. 2013; Whitlock 2006; Wilcox et al. 2012). Disclosure of NSSI is also more likely among people who endorse social-communicative functions of NSSI (Armiento et al. 2014). Unfortunately, many of these disclosures result in only minimal acknowledgment of the NSSI, and conversations that follow are largely rated as unhelpful (Muehlenkamp et al. 2013; Sutherland et al. 2013).

Parents also report that they were often aware of their children's NSSI before their adolescents disclosed it (Oldershaw et al. 2008). Unsurprisingly given the stigma that often surrounds NSSI, parents also describe feeling confused, scared, and reluctant about addressing this behavior with their children (ibid.).

To our knowledge, only one prospective study has examined longer-term consequences of NSSI disclosure, showing that adolescents who did *not* disclose their NSSI reported better relationships with their family and friends over three years, compared to adolescents who disclosed their NSSI (Hasking et al. 2015). However, adolescents who disclosed their NSSI *to an adult* experienced more supportive peer relationships, as well as less frequent NSSI, improvements in problem-focused coping, and increases in reasons for living, relative to adolescents who disclosed their NSSI to peers. Because groups were identified based on baseline disclosure status, it remains unclear whether these differences are a function of the disclosure itself, or of group differences.

In addition to documenting the interpersonal reactions to voluntary disclosures, studies also describe the shock and unhelpful focus on physical, rather than emotional, well-being that often occur following unintended discovery of NSSI by others (Klineberg et al. 2013). Encouragingly, however, people who have told someone about their NSSI in the past are more likely to seek professional help later (Hasking et al. 2015), suggesting that there may be long-term benefits to disclosure even if the initial disclosures are not experienced as helpful. It remains unclear, however, whether people tend to disclose a general history of NSSI (e.g., "I sometimes did/do this") or disclose specific and recent instances of NSSI (e.g., "I did this today/this week"), and how the nature of disclosure or discovery influences its effects. Together, studies in this area suggest that caution is warranted in ascribing social-communicative functions to NSSI, given this behavior often remains hidden.

Can Micro-Longitudinal Methods Test These Assumptions?

While the aforementioned research provides some insight into the tenability of the assumptions of social-communicative models of NSSI, it is less informative regarding the day-to-day antecedents and consequences of specific episodes of NSSI. Unfortunately, studying the immediate precipitants and consequences of NSSI has long posed a challenge to researchers. Much of the research on NSSI has relied on retrospective accounts, which are limited by a participant's ability to recall past NSSI incidents, identify and label possible causes or consequences, and the influence of constructive meaning making that may have occurred since the episode in question (e.g., Klineberg et al. 2013).

Understanding precipitants and consequences of NSSI would ideally be facilitated via direct observations of the behavior, consistent with the behavior analytic approach used to assess and reduce self-injury in developmental disabilities (e.g., Gaylord-Ross et al. 1980; Luiselli et al. 1992). Obtaining direct observations of NSSI poses clear practical and ethical challenges. In the following section, we will describe how micro-longitudinal methods can address gaps in the research and will describe five exemplar studies to illustrate this approach.

MICRO-LONGITUDINAL METHODS—A BRIEF PRIMER

Micro-longitudinal methods use repeated observations of a person as he or she goes about his or her everyday life to understand contingencies that shape behavior. In recent years, the growing use of micro-longitudinal methods in psychological research has moved observation from clinical settings and research labs to individuals' daily experiences. However, researchers new to these methods may encounter several points of confusion on their initial explorations of this literature.

The first potential area of confusion concerns the terminology of the field. "Micro-longitudinal methods" encompass several distinct, but related, methods, and these methods are, in turn, known by numerous names: "experience sampling" (Csikszentmihalyi et al. 1977), "ecological momentary assessment" (EMA) (Stone and Shiffman 1994), "ambulatory monitoring" (Fahrenberg and Myrtek 1996), "daily diaries" (Bolger et al. 2003), "real-time data capture" (Stone et al. 2007), and "intensive longitudinal methods" (Bolger and Laurenceau 2013). All of these terms refer to research designs that share three essential features: They observe individuals in naturalistic settings (as opposed to a lab or clinic), the observations focus on recent or current states and events, and observations are frequently repeated to assess changes in context and behavior. In other words, micro-longitudinal methods involve the repeated observation of individuals' current states as they go about their daily lives.

Ideally, micro-longitudinal studies are designed so that observations are unobtrusive and comprehensive enough to provide a picture of the individual's usual behavior in context. Relationships between theoretically important contexts (e.g., a certain emotional state, spending time in a specific location, or having a particular type of social interaction) and behavior can then be probed statistically, allowing the researcher to determine contingencies that promote or deter a behavior. Because of these features, micro-longitudinal methods are especially well-suited to testing functional theories such as the social-communicative model of NSSI described above.

Within the micro-longitudinal omnibus, a second potential point of confusion concerns variations in study scope and design. For instance, a micro-longitudinal study might collect observations once per day (i.e., daily diary methods), several times per day (i.e., ecological momentary assessment [EMA]), in response to specific events (i.e., event-contingent recording), on a fixed schedule (i.e., interval-contingent recordings), or according to a random plan (i.e., signal-contingent recordings). Observation can rely on participants' self-reports of their subjective states (e.g., current mood), include physiological measures (e.g., salivary samples, continuous heart rate monitoring), or include other objective measures of a person's context or behavior (e.g., acoustic recordings; geo-locations). Technologies used to collect these observations range from pen and paper packets to sophisticated wireless technologies that can be worn on wrists, inside clothes, or mounted in the environment (see, for example, Goodwin 2008).

Deciding which methods should be used depends on the research question, the constructs of interest, the hypothesized temporal dynamics of the contingencies and their relationships, and how these constructs can be most reliably and validly assessed. General principles for designing a micro-longitudinal study are described later in this chapter. For now, it will be helpful to simply acknowledge that researchers have considerable freedom in designing their studies, and study design will have important implications for whether the data will be useful in answering certain types of questions. Most design decisions come with trade-offs such as minimizing burden on participants versus ensuring reports are as inclusive and comprehensive as possible.

A third potential point of confusion concerns the types of statistical analyses that are commonly used to handle data generated by micro-longitudinal studies which are unique in two ways. First, repeated observations generate data that are autocorrelated and violate the assumption of independence that underlies many common statistical tests. Second, these studies can be time-consuming or inconvenient for participants to complete, and so missed reports are common. Both of these are common problems in time-series data and require special considerations to select analytic methods that will generate accurate, unbiased results.

A detailed review of data analytic techniques that are appropriate to micro-longitudinal studies is beyond the scope of this chapter—for excellent coverage of this topic, see Mehl and Conner's (2013) *Handbook of Research Methods for Studying Daily Life* and Singer and Willett's (2003) *Applied Longitudinal Data Analysis: Modeling Change and Event Occurrence*. For our purposes, we wish only to note that readers are likely to encounter a set of analytic techniques called "multilevel," "hierarchical," or "growth" models in this literature, and some familiarity with these techniques may be helpful in understanding the conclusions that researchers draw from their data. We recommend additional resources later in this chapter for beginning analysts who wish to familiarize themselves with these frameworks.

Regardless of the specifics of the design and analyses, micro-longitudinal methods offer several unique methodological advantages. First, they focus on naturalistic patterns of daily living, enhancing the ecological validity of resulting observations. Second, because observations are collected close in time to the phenomenon of interest (e.g., ratings of current mood, logs of activities or social interactions in the past two hours), they reduce well-known biases associated with retrospective and aggregated reports (Bradburn et al. 1987; Nisbett and Wilson 1977; Schacter 1999). Third, they generate repeated observations of the same person over time, making them ideally suited to examining idiographic, within-person processes. Fourth, unlike cross-sectional designs, micro-longitudinal studies can describe and test the sequencing of events, providing key evidence when evaluating potential causal relationships between variables.

MICRO-LONGITUDINAL STUDIES OF THE SOCIAL-COMMUNICATIVE FUNCTIONS OF NSSI IN EVERYDAY LIFE

Despite the relatively nascent state of these methods, micro-longitudinal studies are becoming increasingly common and have already yielded important information regarding the frequency, features, and contexts of NSSI. For instance, given that the most commonly and strongly self-reported function of NSSI is a desire to relieve negative emotional states (Klonsky 2007), several micro-longitudinal studies have sought to clarify the emotional contexts of NSSI.

So far, micro-longitudinal studies suggest that negative affect rises in the hours prior to NSSI and then gradually declines following engagement in NSSI (Andrewes et al. 2017; Armey et al. 2011; Muehlenkamp et al. 2009; Snir et al. 2015). Similarly, positive affect has been shown to decline in the hours before NSSI and then gradually rise following the behavior (Armey et al. 2011; Muehlenkamp et al. 2009). In other words, micro-longitudinal studies support people's perceptions that NSSI helps them to feel better (less negative and more positive).

Although this pattern of findings is consistent with an emotion regulation function of NSSI, one surprising aspect of the findings is the time course over which negative emotions are alleviated and positive emotions resume. In contrast to the assumption that NSSI provides immediate relief from negative emotions, micro-longitudinal studies reveal a much more gradual change in negative emotion which can take ten or more hours to return to its pre-NSSI level (Armey et al. 2011; Snir et al. 2015). Moreover, at least one study has failed to find evidence for a decline in negative affect following NSSI (Houben et al. 2017). This has led some researchers to question whether additional contingencies might be promoting NSSI, such as stabilization (rather than reductions) of negative affect (Vansteelandt et al. 2017), production of positive emotional states (Selby et al. 2014), or regulation of interpersonal contexts (Snir et al. 2015; Turner 2016).

Below, we will describe five illustrative studies that shed light on possible social-communicative functions of NSSI using micro-longitudinal methods. These studies were selected because each one illustrates a unique way of assessing social-communicative functions of NSSI and has advanced our understanding of these models. We hope these examples will show how micro-longitudinal methods can be used to probe functional models and will also provide a summary of important recent findings in this area.

Exemplar Study 1: Do Interpersonal Stressors Commonly Precede NSSI?

One of the earliest micro-longitudinal studies of NSSI was conducted by Nock et al. (2009) who enrolled a cohort of thirty adolescents (87% female), aged twelve to nineteen, each of whom had thought about or engaged in NSSI within the past two weeks. Participants completed two surveys at semi-random intervals through the day and were also instructed to self-initiate a survey whenever they experienced self-destructive thoughts or behaviors. The monitoring continued for fourteen days using a personal digital assistant (PDA). This study captured a total of 344 NSSI thoughts and 104 NSSI behaviors.

Results showed that NSSI behavior was more likely to occur when NSSI thoughts were rated as intense and brief and when the adolescent was alone when the NSSI thoughts began. However, NSSI thoughts also occurred in interpersonal contexts, specifically, when adolescents were with peers, close friends, immediate family, or strangers.

Consistent with retrospective self-report studies, the daily surveys showed that social-communicative functions of NSSI were rarely endorsed relative to emotion relief functions and were viewed as the primary motive for NSSI on fewer than 15 percent of NSSI occasions. However, in line with the notion that social-communicative functions might be under-reported in self-reports—but nonetheless, play an important role in NSSI—multilevel analyses showed that NSSI was significantly more likely to occur when thoughts of NSSI were preceded by feelings of rejection, anger or hatred toward oneself, numbness, or anger toward others.

On the other hand, feeling sad when NSSI thoughts began predicted significantly lower odds of engaging in NSSI, and feeling scared, anxious, or overwhelmed were unassociated with subsequent NSSI behavior. In other words, despite adolescents' self-reports that they engaged in NSSI in order to escape anxiety, sadness, anger, and aversive thoughts and memories, statistical evidence suggests that affective states most strongly predictive of engaging in NSSI are often interpersonally oriented, that is, feeling rejected or feeling angry at others (in addition to feelings of intense self-criticism, shame, or numbness). Moreover, NSSI thoughts were commonly preceded by interpersonal stressors such as arguments or conflict, rejection, criticism or insults, and, in rare cases, encouragement by others to engage in NSSI. Nevertheless, intrapersonal stressors such as worry and upsetting memories were also endorsed. Finally, interpersonally oriented coping strategies (i.e., talking to someone) were the second most common method of *avoiding* acting on NSSI thoughts, superseded only by distraction (i.e., thinking about something else).

Together, these findings illuminate important interpersonal precursors to day-to-day experiences of NSSI. Consistent with social-communicative models of NSSI, these findings showed that interpersonal stressors and interpersonally oriented emotions may serve as triggers for NSSI and that adolescents often use interpersonal strategies to cope with NSSI thoughts, despite the fact that social-communicative functions are rarely explicitly endorsed. This study focused primarily on antecedents to NSSI and provided less information about the interpersonal consequences of NSSI. What remained unanswered, therefore, was whether NSSI effectively modifies interpersonal distress, for instance, by reducing feelings of rejection or by increasing feelings of support.

Exemplar Study 2: Does NSSI Alleviate Interpersonal Distress?

Snir et al. (2015) sought to further probe whether people's explicit, self-reported motives for NSSI matched with the emotional and social contingencies observed before and after NSSI using micro-longitudinal methods. These researchers recruited 152 adults from community and clinical settings. About one-third of the sample met DSM-IV diagnostic criteria for borderline personality disorder, about one-third met diagnostic criteria for avoidant personality disorder, and about one-third did not meet criteria for any psychiatric disorder in the past year. Participants completed five semi-randomly scheduled reports of their current emotions, interpersonal experiences, and NSSI urges and behaviors per day using a PDA over a period of twenty-one days. Of the total sample, twenty-nine participants reported at least one act of NSSI during the study period, and twenty-seven reported at least one NSSI urge.

What did this study teach us about the differences between explicit (self-report) and inferred (statistically derived) motives for NSSI? With respect to explicit motives, the most commonly endorsed function of NSSI acts was to relieve negative emotions, followed closely by generating feelings and punishing oneself. Interpersonal functions such as avoiding others and communicating distress were rarely endorsed by explicit self-report; however, a closer examination of the emotional and interpersonal antecedents and consequences of NSSI gives a fuller picture of possible social-communicative functions. By comparing 20-hour windows surrounding acts of NSSI with 20-hour windows on days without NSSI, Snir and colleagues were able to show that feelings of dissociation and perceived rejection/isolation significantly increased in the hours leading up to NSSI and gradually, but significantly, declined following the behavior. A similar pattern was not observed during comparison periods without NSSI.

Among participants with avoidant personality disorder, NSSI was also preceded by increases in self-devaluation and interpersonally avoidant behaviors and followed by a decline in these experiences several hours after NSSI occurred. The authors interpret these results as providing evidence that NSSI can help regulate not only internally-oriented emotional states such as numbness or dissociation but can also help an individual meet interpersonal needs by reducing feelings of rejection or isolation. Moreover, they note the discrepancy between why participants said they engaged in NSSI (i.e., to relieve general negative emotion) and what actually changed following the behavior (i.e., they felt less numb and less alone or rejected).

Although disclosures and reactions to NSSI were not explicitly examined in this study, the authors conclude that something about NSSI behavior may help an individual feel closer to others. Whether the increase in closeness is a direct consequence of the behavior (e.g., NSSI is disclosed to others who then provide soothing or support) or an indirect consequence of the behavior (e.g., NSSI allows the person to more clearly communicate his or her needs or disrupts ruminative cycles that interfere with communication) is still unclear.

Exemplar Study 3: Do the Consequences of NSSI Depend on Whether Other People Know About the Behavior?

Turner et al. (2016) used a daily diary study to examine whether the antecedents and consequences of NSSI depend on whether NSSI is disclosed/discovered. Participants in this study were sixty young adults (85% female), aged eighteen to thirty-five, with recent (past year) and repeated (10+ lifetime episodes of NSSI) histories of NSSI. All participants endorsed thoughts about or engagement in NSSI in the two weeks prior to study enrolment.

To examine interpersonal antecedents and consequences on NSSI, participants completed a single, retrospective online report detailing their experiences each day for fourteen consecutive days. Within each report, participants were asked to describe their encounters with friends, family, and romantic partners and to rate how supportive these interactions had been. Participants also reported whether they had experienced various types of interpersonal stressors and rated their mood throughout the day in three retrospective periods (morning, afternoon, and evening).

With respect to antecedents of NSSI, results showed that interpersonal stressors were associated with stronger NSSI urges and greater likelihood of engaging in NSSI the same day. The diaries also showed that when NSSI behaviors that had been revealed to others—either because the participant disclosed this behavior or because it was unintentionally discovered—the behavior was followed by increases in the perceived supportiveness of interactions the following day. Moreover, these increases in perceived support that followed NSSI were associated with significantly stronger NSSI urges and a sixfold increase in odds of engaging in NSSI, compared to perceived support that did not follow NSSI.

These results provide the most direct test of the social-communicative function of NSSI using micro-longitudinal data yet, supporting each of the three assumptions outlined in the previous section: that NSSI is occasioned by interpersonal needs (i.e., heightened interpersonal conflict or other interpersonal stressors), that NSSI can promote desirable changes in the interpersonal environment (i.e., increases in perceived support), and that these desirable consequences are most apparent when other people are aware of the NSSI behavior. Consistent with the four-function model (Nock and Prinstein 2004), this study also supports the reinforcing nature of social-communicative functions, showing that increases in perceived support following NSSI are associated with increased urges for and engagement in NSSI.

Exemplar Studies 4 and 5: How and Why Might NSSI Help Meet Interpersonal Needs?

Up to this point, the studies we've discussed have examined the antecedents and consequences of NSSI in order to probe possible social-communicative functions of the behavior. Evidence from Nock et al. (2009), Snir et al. (2015) and Turner et al. (2016) supports the notion that NSSI often occurs in response to interpersonal stressors and modifies these aversive interpersonal experiences, either by decreasing feelings of rejection or by increasing perceptions of social support. Importantly, there is some evidence that these shifts may only occur when other people are aware of recent NSSI behavior and that these shifts increase cravings for and engagement in subsequent NSSI.

A persistent question is why some people use NSSI to meet interpersonal needs in the first place. After all, there are many other behaviors that could signal distress, communicate a need for support, or repair interpersonal conflict (see Nock 2008). A more recent line of micro-longitudinal research has examined the daily social experiences of people who engage in NSSI in order to understand why they may be vulnerable to this behavior. We will briefly describe two recent studies illustrating this approach to underscore the range in questions that can be addressed in micro-longitudinal work.

Using the same sample and design described above, Turner et al. (2017) compared daily experiences of interpersonal contact, conflict, and support, as well as use of social support to cope with distress among the sixty young adults with NSSI and fifty-six young adults (70% female) with no history of NSSI. Compared to people with no experience of NSSI, people who engaged in NSSI reported that they had less contact with their peers and rated their peer interactions as less supportive. Relative to people without NSSI, they had less contact with their family members and more contact with their romantic partners, but there were no differences in how supportive they rated these interactions. Overall, this suggests that people with NSSI may rely on a more limited social network for support. Given that people with NSSI were also more likely to seek support to cope with distress, compared to people who didn't engage in NSSI, their relationships may be more frequently taxed, which could exacerbate stress.

In a similar study, Santangelo et al. (2017) compared the social experiences of twenty-six female adolescents (aged thirteen to eighteen) with recent (past year) NSSI and twenty age-matched adolescents with no history of NSSI. For two consecutive weekends, participants provided hourly ratings of their mood, their relationship with their mother, and their relationship with their best friend. Results showed that, relative to adolescents with no history of NSSI, adolescents with a history of NSSI rated themselves as feeling less attached to their mothers and best friends. These ratings were also more variable, however, indicating that youth with a history of NSSI were more likely to experience shifts in how they viewed their relationships with others (e.g., going from feeling close to distant, or positive to negative, in a short period of time).

Together, results from these final studies illustrate how micro-longitudinal methods can help characterize the interpersonal experiences of people who engage in NSSI. An important next step in this line of research is examining whether differences in the quality and quantity of these interpersonal experiences precede (as a potential cause) or follow (as a potential consequence) the onset of NSSI.

DESIGN CONSIDERATION AND RESOURCES FOR MICRO-LONGITUDINAL STUDIES OF NSSI

The five studies described above illustrate the utility of micro-longitudinal methods for testing many of the assumptions underlying social-communicative models of NSSI. Hopefully, this discussion has persuaded some readers to consider incorporating such methods into their research or clinical work. Below, we provide a few "best practice" recommendations for beginning NSSI researchers to ensure future studies are maximally informative.

1) Consider the Frequency of Assessment

The timing and number of assessments each day should be informed by how often the constructs of interest are expected to vary and how accurately they can be recalled after the fact. For instance, perceptions of social interactions might be most easily rated soon after the interaction, requiring the option for participants to make several ratings per day, while major stressors such as arguments or NSSI acts may easily be recalled and described in a single, end-of-day report. Overall, the decision about how often to ask people to make ratings or reports should balance accuracy and informativeness of reports with minimization of participant burden and reactivity. Studies that seek to examine functions of NSSI are advised to use multiple reports per day to allow for accurate sequencing of antecedents and consequences of behavior as well as investigation of non-linear trends that are commonly identified (e.g., Muehlenkamp et al. 2009; Snir et al. 2015).

2) Balance Breadth, Depth and Validity in Measure Selection

Due to the frequency of assessments, many micro-longitudinal studies use brief scales, or even a single item, to assess constructs of interest. There are notable benefits and drawbacks of this approach. Given that measurement error is an inherent feature of self-reported measurement of psychological constructs, researchers are advised to choose multi-item scales where possible and to carefully assess the reliability and validity of the measure. Ideally, the measure will have a high degree of between- and within-person reliability, but will also be sensitive to change (see, for example, Wilhelm and Schoebi 2007). Fortunately, the number of measures that have been specifically validated for use in micro-longitudinal research is rapidly growing. For an excellent discussion of psychometric theory as applied to micro-longitudinal designs, readers may wish to consult Shrout and Lane (2011).

3) Consider Using Technologies that Makes Participation Easier

With the rise of smartphones and wearables, ready-made applications to facilitate micro-longitudinal studies are now widely available; however, researchers and clinicians should pay careful attention to privacy and confidentiality policies and the degree of testing or validation when choosing third-party apps. As others have noted, many apps are marketed with bold claims regarding their efficacy without sufficient evidence (Larsen et al. 2019). Features that researchers may wish to seek include automatic date/time stamping, flexible prompt scheduling, options to alert research staff if a certain type of response is received (e.g., participants who endorse serious suicidal thoughts), dashboards that allow real-time compliance monitoring, and user features that can promote compliance (e.g., graphical displays of responses, incentives or reminders, or options to pause data collection).

4) Provide Appropriate Incentives

All of the micro-longitudinal studies described in this paper offered monetary compensation to participants ranging from around $60 to $120, varying as a function of study length, report frequency and participant compliance (i.e., how many reports were completed). This generally seems to be an effective strategy for minimizing missing data. However, researchers must take care not to offer payment that could be coercive, especially when working with younger participants. Researchers operating on a limited budget might want to consider non-monetary incentives that could be offered to encourage compliance, for instance offering NSSI resources or individualized feedback regarding data provided—assuming the researcher has appropriate qualifications to interpret the data and provide such feedback in a way that does not go beyond the scope or implications of the information collected.

5) Consider Your Ethical Obligations to Participants

Given that people who engage in NSSI may be considered a vulnerable population, protocols for risk assessment and management should be defined before starting data collection. For instance, under what conditions will the investigator contact participants during data collection, if ever? At what point might lack of response indicate a participant has dropped out of the study, and what will happen if that occurs? If a participant requires urgent medical or psychological assistance during the study, who should he or she contact, and how will the researcher facilitate these contacts, if at all? Guidelines for conducting research with populations who engage in NSSI are provided in Lloyd-Richardson et al. (2015), and examples of approved protocols for micro-longitudinal studies that incorporate smartphones, passive sensors, and ambulatory monitories may be found on the Connected and Open Research Ethics (CORE) website (https://thecore-platform.ucsd.edu/resources).

6) Use Appropriate Analyses to Handle Data

As described above, the appropriate data analytic plan will depend on the research question and structure of the data. However, researchers who seek to understand the functions of NSSI are advised to include occasions with *and without* NSSI in analyses because focusing only on moments when the behavior has occurred can be misleading (Paty et al. 1992). For instance, declining loneliness following NSSI could reflect a consequence of NSSI, or it could reflect a natural return to baseline (or regression to the mean) following extreme responses. The need to capture both types of reports should inform sample size, inclusion criteria, and study duration. Limitations related to the generalizability of findings related to these design decisions should be acknowledged. Further recommended resources are provided at the end of this chapter.

FUTURE DIRECTIONS AND CONCLUSIONS

Researchers have advocated that, when it comes to understanding naturalistic occurrence of suicidal thoughts and behaviors, larger and longer micro-longitudinal studies are urgently needed (Kleiman and Nock 2018). We believe the same is true for studies of NSSI. So far, sample sizes have been relatively small (Ns = 26 to 60), and the longest micro-longitudinal study (Snir et al. 2015) lasted only three weeks. Understanding contingencies that promote and deter NSSI will require observing many occasions on which this behavior does and does not occur, elucidating between- and within-person processes that contribute to occurrence, and understanding how these dynamics can change as a function of time and history (e.g., whether a person has newly commenced NSSI or has been engaging in the behavior for years). Given that adolescents' and parents' perceptions regarding NSSI do not always align (e.g., Baetens et al. 2014; Oldershaw et al. 2008), the inclusion of multiple informants in our studies will help us get a fuller picture of how NSSI behavior impacts relationships.

As mentioned above, rapidly evolving technologies permit unprecedented variety in the types of data that can now be collected in "real-time." Wearable sensors can monitor physiological arousal and physical activity (Bussmann et al. 2009; Wilhelm et al. 2012). Acoustic sensors can capture duration and emotional valence of interactions (Mehl and Robbins 2012). Harnessing these technologies could provide an opportunity to further expand our understanding of social-communicative functions of NSSI in daily life beyond the information available through self-reports.

In summary, micro-longitudinal methods are well-suited to testing the foundational assumptions of social-communicative functional models of NSSI—that is, that interpersonal contingencies such as conflict, rejection and unwanted bids for connection increase the probability that the behavior will occur, that the behavior can modify the interpersonal environment in desirable ways, and that the efficiency of the behavior in producing these changes depends on the extent to which NSSI is directly or indirectly communicated.

While prospective studies of interpersonal contingencies over months and years have yielded mixed results, particularly for the second and third assumptions, we would argue that social-communicative functions are likely to play out over a shorter time course (e.g., minutes, hours, or days). Thus, greater clarity may be reached by expanding the use of micro-longitudinal designs to complement traditional longitudinal methods. However, it is worth noting that very few micro-longitudinal studies have yet examined the social-communicative functions of NSSI, and replication is urgently needed if we are to put stock in the current findings. Expansion of these methods will help understand what is being communicated by NSSI, when and with whom it is communicated, and how we can be most helpful to individuals who struggle with this behavior.

Recommended Resources

- Bolger, Niall, and Jean-Philippe Laurenceau. *Intensive Longitudinal Methods: An Introduction to Diary and Experience Sampling Research.* New York, NY: Guilford Press, 2013.
- Mehl, Matthias R., and Tamlin S. Conner. *Handbook of Research Methods for Studying Daily Life.* New York, NY: Guilford Press, 2012.
- Singer, Judith D., and John B. Willett. *Applied Longitudinal Data Analysis.* New York, NY: Oxford University Press, 2003.

REFERENCES

Andover, Margaret S., and Blair W. Morris. "Expanding and Clarifying the Role of Emotion Regulation in Nonsuicidal Self-Injury." *Canadian Journal of Psychiatry* 59, no. 11 (2014): 569–575.

Andrewes, Holly E., Carol Hulbert, Susan M. Cotton, Jennifer Betts, and Andrew M. Chanen. "An Ecological Momentary Assessment Investigation of Complex and Conflicting Emotions in Youth with Borderline Personality Disorder." *Psychiatry Research* 252 (2017): 102–110. doi:10.1016/j.psychres.2017.01.100

Armey, Michael F., Janis H. Crowther, and Ivan W. Miller. "Changes in Ecological Momentary Assessment Reported Affect Associated with Episodes of Nonsuicidal Self-Injury." *Behavior Therapy* 42, no. 4 (2011): 579–588. doi:10.1016/j.beth.2011.01.002

Baetens, Imke, Laurence Claes, Patrick Onghena, Hans Grietens, Karla Van Leeuwen, Ciska Pieters, Jan R. Wiersema, and James W. Griffith. "Non-Suicidal Self-Injury in Adolescence: A Longitudinal Study of the Relationship Between NSSI, Psychological Distress and Perceived Parenting." *Journal of Adolescence* 37, no. 6 (2014): 817–826. doi:10.1016/j.adolescence.2014.05.010

Baetens, Imke, Laurence Claes, Patrick Onghena, Hans Grietens, Karla Van Leeuwen, Ciska Pieters, Jan R. Wiersema, and James W. Griffith. "The Effects of Nonsuicidal Self-Injury on Parenting Behaviors: A Longitudinal Analyses of the Perspective of the Parent." *Child and Adolescent Psychiatry and Mental Health* 9 (2015): 24. doi:10.1186/s13034-015-0059-2

Bolger, Niall, Angelina Davis, and Eshkol Rafaeli. "Diary Methods: Capturing Life as it is Lived." *Annual Review of Psychology* 54 (2003): 579–616. doi:10.1146/annurev.psych.54.101601.145030

Bolger, Niall, and Jean-Philippe Laurenceau. *Intensive Longitudinal Methods: An Introduction to Diary and Experience Sampling Research*. New York, NY: Guilford Press, 2013.

Bowes, Lucy, Rebecca Carnegie, Rebecca Pearson, Becky Mars, Lucy Biddle, Barbara Maughan, Glyn Lewis, Charles Fernylough, and Jon Heron. "Risk of Depression and Self-Harm in Teenagers Identifying with Goth Subculture: A Longitudinal Cohort Study." *The Lancet Psychiatry* 2, no. 9 (2015): 793–800. doi:10.1016/S2215-0366(15)00164-9

Bradburn, N. M., L. J. Rips, and S. K. Shevell. "Answering Autobiographical Questions: The Impact of Memory and Inference on Surveys." *Science (New York, N.Y.)* 236, no. 4798 (1987): 157–161.

Briere, John, and Eliana Gil. "Self-Mutilation in Clinical and General Population Samples: Prevalence, Correlates, and Functions." *American Journal of Orthopsychiatry* 68, no. 4 (1998): 609–620. doi:10.1037/h0080369

Burke, T. A., B. A. Ammerman, J. L. Hamilton, and L. B. Alloy. "Impact of Non-Suicidal Self-Injury Scale: Initial Psychometric Validation." *Cognitive Therapy and Research* 41, no. 1 (2017): 130–142. doi:10.1007/s10608-016-9806-9

Burke, Taylor A., Jessica L. Hamilton, Lyn Y. Abramson, and Lauren B. Alloy. "Non-Suicidal Self-Injury Prospectively Predicts Interpersonal Stressful Life Events and Depressive Symptoms Among Adolescent Girls." *Psychiatry Research* 228, no. 3 (2015): 416–424. doi:10.1016/j.psychres.2015.06.021

Bussmann, Johannes B. J., Ulrich W. Ebner-Priemer, and Jochen Fahrenberg. "Ambulatory Activity Monitoring: Progress in Measurement of Activity, Posture, and Specific Motion Patterns in Daily Life." *European Psychologist* 14, no. 2 (2009): 142–152. doi:10.1027/1016-9040.14.2.142

Chapman, Alexander L., Kim L. Gratz, and Milton Z. Brown. "Solving the Puzzle of Deliberate Self-Harm: The Experiential Avoidance Model." *Behavior Research and Therapy* 44, no. 3 (2006): 371–394. doi:10.1016/j.brat.2005.03.005

Christoffersen, Mogens Nygaard, Bo Møhl, Diana DePanfilis, and Katrine S. Vammen. "Non-Suicidal Self-Injury—Does Social Support Make a Difference? An Epidemiological Investigation of a Danish National Sample." *Child Abuse and Neglect* 44 (2015): 106–116. doi:10.1016/j.chiabu.2014.10.023

Claes, Laurence, Adinda Houben, Walter Vandereycken, Patricia Bijttebier, and Jennifer Muehlenkamp. "Brief Report: The Association Between Non-Suicidal Self-Injury, Self-Concept and Acquaintance with Self-Injurious Peers in a Sample of Adolescents." *Journal of Adolescence* 33, no. 5 (2010): 775–778. doi:10.1016/j.adolescence.2009.10.012

Claes, Laurence, Koen Luyckx, Imke Baetens, Monique Van de Ven, and Cilia Witteman. "Bullying and Victimization, Depressive Mood, and Non-Suicidal Self-Injury in Adolescents: The Moderating Role of Parental Support." *Journal of Child and Family Studies* 24, no. 11 (2015): 3363–3371. doi:10.1007/s10826-015-0138-2

Csikszentmihalyi, Mihaly, Reed Larson, and Suzanne Prescott. "The Ecology of Adolescent Activity and Experience." *Journal of Youth and Adolescence* 6, no. 3 (1977): 281–294. doi:10.1007/BF02138940

Di Pierro, Rossella, Irene Sarno, Sara Perego, Marcello Gallucci, and Fabio Madeddu. "Adolescent Nonsuicidal Self-Injury: The Effects of Personality Traits, Family Relationships and Maltreatment on the Presence and Severity of Behaviors." *European Child and Adolescent Psychiatry* 21, no. 9 (2012): 511–520. doi:10.1007/s00787-012-0289-2

Fahrenberg, Jochen, and Michael Myrtek (Eds.). *Ambulatory Assessment: Computer-Assisted Psychological and Psychophysiological Methods in Monitoring and Field Studies.* Seattle, WA: Hogrefe and Huber, 1996.

Favazza, Armondo R. "Why Patients Mutilate Themselves." *Hospital and Community Psychiatry* 40 (1989): 137–145.

Favazza, Armondo R., and Richard J. Rosenthal. "Diagnostic Issues in Self-Mutilation." *Hospital and Community Psychiatry* 44, no. 2 (1993): 134–140.

Fox, Kathryn R., Jill M. Hooley, Diana M. Y. Smith, Jessica D. Ribeiro, Xieyining Huang, Matthew K. Nock, and Joseph C. Franklin. "Self-Injurious Thoughts and Behaviors May Be More Common and Severe among People Identifying as a Sexual Minority." *Behavior Therapy* 49, no. 5 (2017): 768–780. doi:10.1016/j.beth.2017.11.009

Fox, Kathryn R., Joseph C. Franklin, Jessica D. Ribeiro, Evan M. Kleiman, Kate H. Bentley, and Matthem K. Nock. "Meta-Analysis of Risk Factors for Nonsuicidal Self-Injury." *Clinical Psychology Review* 42 (2015): 156–167. doi:10.1016/j.cpr.2015.09.002

Gaylord-Ross, Robert J., Marian Weeks, and Carol Lipner. "An Analysis of Antecedent, Response, and Consequence Events in the Treatment of Self-Injurious Behavior." *Education and Training of the Mentally Retarded* 15, no. 1 (1980): 35–42. Division on Autism and Developmental Disabilities. doi:10.2307/23889350

Giletta, Matteo, Ron H. J. Scholte, Rutger C. M. E. Engels, Silvia Ciairano, and Mitchell J. Prinstein. "Adolescent Non-Suicidal Self-Injury: A Cross-National Study of Community Samples from Italy, the Netherlands and the United States." *Psychiatry Research* 197, no. 1–2 (2012): 66–72. doi:10.1016/j.psychres.2012.02.009

Goodwin, Matthew S. "Enhancing and Accelerating the Pace of Autism Research and Treatment: The Promise of Developing Innovative Technology." *Focus on Autism and Other Developmental Disabilities* 23, no. 2 (2008): 125–128. doi:10.1177/1088357608316678

Gratz, Kim L. "Risk Factors for and Functions of Deliberate Self-Harm: An Empirical and Conceptual Review." *Clinical Psychology: Science and Practice* 10, no. 2 (2003): 192–205. doi:10.1093/clipsy/bpg022

Groschwitz, Rebecca C., and Paul L. Plener. "The Neurobiology of Non-Suicidal Self-Injury (NSSI): A Review." *Suicidology Online* 3 (2012): 24–32.

Guerry, John D., and Mitchell J. Prinstein. "Longitudinal Prediction of Adolescent Nonsuicidal Self-Injury: Examination of a Cognitive Vulnerability-Stress Model." *Journal of Clinical Child and Adolescent Psychology: The Official Journal for the Society of Clinical Child and Adolescent Psychology, American Psychological Association, Division* 39, no. 1 (2010): 77–89. doi:10.1080/15374410903401195

Hankin, Benjamin L., Andrea L. Barrocas, Jami F. Young, Brett Haberstick, and Andrea Smolen. "5-HTTLPR×Interpersonal Stress Interaction and Nonsuicidal Self-Injury in General Community Sample of Youth." *Psychiatry Research* 225, no. 3 (2014): 609–612. doi:10.1016/j.psychres.2014.11.037

Hankin, Benjamin L., and John R. Z. Abela. "Nonsuicidal Self-Injury in Adolescence: Prospective Rates and Risk factors in a 2½ Year Longitudinal Study." *Psychiatry Research* 186, no. 1 (2011): 65–70. doi:10.1016/j.psychres.2010.07.056

Hasking, Penelope, Clare S. Rees, Graham Martin, and Jessie Quigley. "What Happens When You Tell Someone You Self-Injure? The Effects of Disclosing NSSI to Adults and Peers." *BMC Public Health* 15 (2015): 1039. doi:10.1186/s12889-015-2383-0

Heath, Nancy L., Shana Ross, Jessica R. Toste, Alison Charlebois, and Tatiana Nedecheva. "Retrospective Analysis of Social Factors and Nonsuicidal Self-Injury Among Young adults." *Canadian Journal of Behavioral Science* 41, no. 3 (2009): 180–186. doi:10.1037/a0015732

Heilbron, Nicole, Joseph C. Franklin, John D. Guerry, and Mitchell J. Prinstein. "Social and Ecological Approaches to Understanding Suicidal Behaviors and Nonsuicidal Self-Injury." In *The Oxford Handbook of Suicide and Self-Injury*, edited by Matthew K. Nock, 206–234. New York, NY: Oxford University Press, 2014.

Hilt, Lori M., Christine B. Cha, and Susan Nolen-Hoeksema. "Nonsuicidal Self-Injury in Young Adolescent Girls: Moderators of the Distress-Function Relationship." *Journal of Consulting and Clinical Psychology* 76, no. 1 (2008): 63–71. doi:10.1037/0022-006X.76.1.63

Hilt, Lori M., Matthew K. Nock, Elizabeth E. Lloyd-Richardson, and Mitchell J. Prinstein. "Longitudinal Study of Nonsuicidal Self-Injury Among Young Adolescents: Rates, Correlates, and Preliminary Test of an Interpersonal Model." *The Journal of Early Adolescence* 28, no. 3 (2008): 455–469. doi:10.1177/0272431608316604

Hooley, Jill M., and Joseph C. Franklin. "Why Do People Hurt Themselves? A New Conceptual Model of Nonsuicidal Self-Injury." *Clinical Psychological Science* 6, no. 3 (2018): 428–451. doi:10.1177/2167702617745641

Houben, Marlies, Laurence Claes, Kristof Vansteelandt, Ann Berens, Ellen Sleuwaegen, and Peter Kuppens. "The Emotion Regulation Function of Nonsuicidal Self-Injury: A Momentary Assessment Study in Inpatients with Borderline Personality Disorder Features." *Journal of Abnormal Psychology* 126, no. 1 (2017): 89–95. doi:10.1037/abn0000229

Jacobson, Colleen, and K. Batejan (2014). "Comprehensive Theoretical Models of Nonsuicidal Self-Injury." In *The Oxford Handbook of Suicide and Self-Injury*, edited by Matthew K. Nock. New York: Oxford University Press, 2014. doi:10.1093/oxfordhb/9780195388565.013.0017

Jacobson, Colleen McClain, Ryan M. Hill, Jeremy W. Pettit, and Dima Grozeva. "The Association of Interpersonal and Intrapersonal Emotional Experiences with Non-Suicidal Self-Injury in Young Adults." *Archives of Suicide Research* 19, no. 4 (2015): 401–413. doi:10.1080/13811118.2015.1004492

Keenan, Kate, Alison E. Hipwell, Stephanie D. Stepp, and Kristen Wroblewski. "Testing an Equifinality Model of Nonsuicidal Self-Injury Among Early Adolescent Girls." *Development and Psychopathology* 26, no. 3 (2014): 851–862. doi:10.1017/S0954579414000431

Kerr, Patrick L., Jennifer J. Muehlenkamp, and James M. Turner. "Nonsuicidal Self-Injury: A Review of Current Research for Family Medicine and Primary Care Physicians." *Journal of the American Board of Family Medicine* 23, no. 2 (2010): 240–259. doi:10.3122/jabfm.2010.02.090110

Kim, Kerri L., Grace K. Cushman, Alexandra B. Weissman, Megan E. Puzia, Ezra Wegbreit, Erin B. Tone, Anthony Spiriton, and Daniel P. Dickstein. "Behavioral and Emotional Responses to Interpersonal Stress: A Comparison of Adolescents Engaged in Non-Suicidal Self-Injury to Adolescent Suicide Attempters." *Psychiatry Research* 228, no. 3 (2015): 899–906. doi:10.1016/j.psychres.2015.05.001

Kleiman, Evan M., and Matthew K. Nock. "Real-Time Assessment of Suicidal Thoughts and Behaviors." *Current Opinion in Psychology* 22 (2018): 33–37. doi:10.1016/j.copsyc.2017.07.026

Kleindienst, Nikolaus, Martin Bohus, Petra Ludäscher, Matthias F. Limberger, Katrin Kuenkele, Ulrich W. Ebner-Priemer, Alexander L. Chapman, Markus Reicherzer, Rolf-Dieter Stieglitz, and Christian Schmahl. "Motives for Nonsuicidal Self-Injury Among Women with Borderline Personality Disorder." *Journal of Nervous and Mental Disease* 196, no. 3 (2008): 230–236. doi:10.1097/NMD.0b013e3181663026

Klineberg, Emily, Moira J. Kelly, Stephen A. Stansfeld, and Kamaldeep S. Bhui. "How Do Adolescents Talk About Self-Harm: A Qualitative Study of Disclosure in an Ethnically Diverse Urban Population in England." *BMC Public Health* 13, no. 1 (2013). doi:10.1186/1471-2458-13-572

Klonsky, E. David. "The Functions of Deliberate Self-Injury: A Review of the Evidence." *Clinical Psychology Review* 27, no. 2 (2007): 226–239. doi:10.1016/j.cpr.2006.08.002

Klonsky, E. David. "Non-Suicidal Self Injury in United States Adults: Prevalence, Sociodemographics, Topography and Functions." *Psychological Medicine: A Journal of Research in Psychiatry and the Allied Sciences* 41, no. 9 (2011): 1981–1986.

Klonsky, E. David, Sarah E. Victor, and Boaz Y. Saffer. "Nonsuicidal Self-Injury: What We Know, and What We Need to Know." *Canadian Journal of Psychiatry* 59, no. 11 (2014): 565–568.

Laghi, Fiorenzo, Arriana Terrinoni, Rita Cerutti, Fiorella Fantini, Serena Galosi, Mauro Ferrara, and Frencesca Marina Bosco. "Theory of Mind in Non-Suicidal Self-Injury (NSSI) Adolescents." *Consciousness and Cognition* 43 (2016): 38–47. doi:10.1016/j.concog.2016.05.004

Larsen, Mark Erik, Kit Huckvale, Jennifer Nicholas, John Torous, Louise Birrell, Emily Li, and Bill Reda. "Using Science to Sell Apps: Evaluation of Mental Health App Store Quality." *npj Digital Medicine* 2, no. 18 (2019).

Lewis, Stephen P., and Saba Mehrabkhani. "Every Scar Tells a Story: Insight Into People's Self-Injury Scar Experiences." *Counselling Psychology Quarterly* 29, no. 3 (2016): 296–310. doi:10.1080/09515070.2015.1088431

Linehan, Marsha M. *Cognitive-Behavioral Treatment for Borderline Personality Disorder: The Dialectics of Effective Treatment*. New York, NY: Guilford Press, 1993.

Lloyd-Richardson, Elizabeth E., Stephen P. Lewis, Janis L. Whitlock, Karen Rodham, and Heather T. Schatten. "Research with Adolescents Who Engage in Non-Suicidal Self-Injury: Ethical Considerations and Challenges." *Child and Adolescent Psychiatry and Mental Health* 9, no. 1 (2015): 37. doi:10.1186/s13034-015-0071-6

Luiselli, James K., Johnny L. Matson, and Nirbhay N. Singh. *Self-Injurious Behavior: Analysis, Assessment, and Treatment*. New York, NY: Springer-Verlag, 1992.

Mehl, Matthias R., and Megan L. Robbins. "Naturalistic Observation Sampling: The Electronically Activated Recorder (EAR)." In *Handbook of Research Methods for Studying Daily Life*, edited by Matthias R. Mehl and Tamlin S. Conner, 176–192. New York: Guilford Press, 2012.

Muehlenkamp, Jennifer, Amy Brausch, Katherine Quigley, and Janis Whitlock. "Interpersonal Features and Functions of Nonsuicidal Self-Injury." *Suicide and Life-Threatening Behavior* 43, no. 1 (2013): 67–80. doi:10.1111/j.1943-278X.2012.00128.x

Muehlenkamp, Jennifer J., Laurence Claes, Lindsey Havertape, and Paul L. Plener. "International Prevalence of Adolescent Non-Suicidal Self-Injury and Deliberate Self-Harm." *Child and Adolescent Psychiatry and Mental Health* 6, no. 1 (2012): 10. doi:10.1186/1753-2000-6-10

Muehlenkamp, Jennifer J., Lori M. Hilt, Peter P. Ehlinger, and Taylor McMillan. "Nonsuicidal Self-Injury in Sexual Minority College Students: A Test of Theoretical Integration." *Child and Adolescent Psychiatry and Mental Health* 9 (2015): 16. doi:10.1186/s13034-015-0050-y

Muehlenkamp, Jennifer J., Scott G. Engel, Andrea Wadeson, Ross D. Crosby, Stephen A. Wonderlich, Heather Simonich, and James E. Mitchell. "Emotional States Preceding and Following Acts of Non-Suicidal Self-Injury in Bulimia Nervosa Patients." *Behavior Research and Therapy* 47, no. 1 (2009): 83–87. doi:10.1016/j.brat.2008.10.011

Nisbett, Richard E., and Timothy D. Wilson. "Telling More Than We Can Know: Verbal Reports on Mental Processes." *Psychological Review* 84 (1977): 231–259.

Nock, Matthew K. "Actions Speak Louder Than Words: An Elaborated Theoretical Model of the Social Functions of Self-Injury and Other Harmful Behaviors." *Applied and Preventive Psychology* 12 (2008): 159–168.

Nock, Matthew K. "Why Do People Hurt Themselves? New Insights Into the Nature and Functions of Self-Injury." *Current Directions in Psychological Science* 18, no. 2 (2009): 78–83. doi:10.1111/j.1467-8721.2009.01613.x

Nock, Matthew K., and Mitchell J. Prinstein. "A Functional Approach to the Assessment of Self-Mutilative Behavior." *Journal of Consulting and Clinical Psychology* 72, no. 5 (2004): 885–890. doi:10.1037/0022-006X.72.5.885

Nock, Matthew K., and Mitchell J. Prinstein. "Clinical Features and Behavioral Functions of Adolescent Self-Mutilation." *Journal of Abnormal Psychology* 114 (2005): 140–146.

Nock, Matthew K., Mitchell J. Prinstein, and Sonya K. Sterba. "Revealing the Form and Function of Self-Injurious Thoughts and Behaviors: A Real-Time Ecological Assessment Study Among Adolescents and Young Adults." *Journal of Abnormal Psychology* 118, no. 4 (2009): 816–827. doi:10.1037/a0016948; 10.1037/a0016948.supp (Supplemental)

Nock, Matthew K., and Wendy Berry Mendes. "Physiological Arousal, Distress Tolerance, and Social Problem-Solving Deficits Among Adolescent Self-Injurers." *Journal of Consulting and Clinical Psychology* 76, no. 1 (2008): 28–38. doi:10.1037/0022-006X.76.1.28

Oldershaw, Anna, Clair Richards, Mima Simic, and Ulrike Schmidt. "Parents' Perspectives on Adolescent Self-Harm: Qualitative Study." *The British Journal of Psychiatry* 193, no. 2 (2008): 140–144. doi:10.1192/bjp.bp.107.045930

Paty, Jean, Jon Kassel, and Saul Shiffman. "The Importance of Assessing Base Rates for Clinical Studies: An Example of Stimulus Control of Smoking." In *The Experience of Psychopathology*, edited by M. W. de Vries, 347–352. Cambridge: Cambridge University Press, 2006. doi:10.1017/CBO9780511663246.031

Plener, Paul L., Mark Alroggen, Nestor D. Kapusta, Elmar Brähler, Jorg M. Fegert, and Rebecca C. Groschwitz. "The Prevalence of Nonsuicidal Self-Injury (NSSI) in a Representative Sample of the German Population." *BMC Psychiatry* 16, no. 1 (2016): 353. doi:10.1186/s12888-016-1060-x

Prinstein, Mitchell J. "Introduction to the Special Section on Suicide and Nonsuicidal Self-Injury: A Review of Unique Challenges and Important Directions for Self-Injury Science." *Journal of Consulting and Clinical Psychology* 76, no. 1 (2008): 1–8. doi:10.1037/0022-006X.76.1.1

Rodham, Karen, Jeffrey Gavin, Stephen Lewis, Peter Bandalli, and Jill St. Denis. "The NSSI Paradox: Discussing and Displaying NSSI in an Online Environment." *Deviant Behavior* 37, no. 10 (2016): 1110–1117. doi:10.1080/01639625.2016.1169747

Rosen, Paul, and Barent Walsh. "Relationship Patterns in Episodes of Self-Mutilative Contagion." *The American Journal of Psychiatry* 146 (1989): 656–658.

Rosen, Paul M., and Barent W. Walsh. "Patterns of Contagion in Self-Mutilation Epidemics." *The American Journal of Psychiatry* 146, no. 5 (1989): 656–658.

Rosen, Paul M., Barent W. Walsh, and Sarah A. Rode. "Interpersonal Loss and Self-Mutilation." *Suicide and Life-Threatening Behavior* 20, no. 2 (1990): 177–184.

Rotolone, Cassandra, and Graham Martin. "Giving Up Self-Injury: A Comparison of Everyday Social and Personal Resources in Past Versus Current Self-Injurers." *Archives of Suicide Research* 16 (2012): 147–158. doi:10.1080/13811118.2012.667333

Santangelo, Philip S., Julian Koenig, Vera Funke, Peter Parzer, Franz Resch, Ulrich W. Ebner-Priemer, and Michael Kaess. "Ecological Momentary Assessment of Affective and Interpersonal Instability in Adolescent Non-Suicidal Self-Injury."

Journal of Abnormal Child Psychology 45, no. 7 (2017): 1429–1438. doi:10.1007/s10802-016-0249-2

Schacter, Daniel L. "The Seven Sins of Memory; Insights from Psychology and Cognitive Neuroscience." *The American Psychologist* 54, no. 3 (1999): 182–203.

Selby, Edward A., Matthew K. Nock, and Amy Kranzler. "How Does Self-Injury Feel? Examining Automatic Positive Reinforcement in Adolescent Self-Injurers with Experience Sampling." *Psychiatry Research* 215, no. 2 (2014): 417–423. doi:10.1016/j.psychres.2013.12.005

Serafini, Gianluca, Giovanna Canepa, Giulia Adavastro, Japopo Nebbia, Martino Belvederi Murri, Denise Erbuto, Benedetta Pocai, Andrea Fiorillo, Maurizio Pompili, Eirini Flouri, and Mario Amore. "The Relationship between Childhood Maltreatment and Non-Suicidal Self-Injury: A Systematic Review." *Frontiers in Psychiatry* 8 (2017): 149. doi:10.3389/fpsyt.2017.00149

Shiffman, Saul. "Conceptualizing Analyses of Ecological Momentary Assessment Data." *Nicotine and Tobacco Research: Official Journal of the Society for Research on Nicotine and Tobacco* 16, no. Suppl 2 (2014): S76–S87. doi:10.1093/ntr/ntt195

Shrout, Patrick E., and Sean P. Lane. "Psychometrics." In *Handbook of Research Methods for Studying Daily Life*, edited by M. R. Mehl and T. A. Conner, 302–320. New York, NY: Guilford Press, 2011.

Snir, Avigal, Eshkol Rafaeli, Reuma Gadassi, Kathy Berenson, and Geraldine Downey. "Explicit and Inferred Motives for Nonsuicidal Self-Injurious Acts and Urges in Borderline and Avoidant Personality Disorders." *Personality Disorders: Theory, Research, and Treatment* 6, no. 3 (2015): 267–277. doi:10.1037/per0000104

Stone, Arthur A., and Saul Shiffman. "Ecological Momentary Assessment (EMA) in Behavorial Medicine." *Annals of Behavioral Medicine* 16, no. 3 (1994): 199–202.

Stone, Arthur A., Saul Shiffman, Audie Atienza, and Linda Nebeling. *The Science of Real-Time Data Capture: Self-Reports in Health Research*. Oxford, England: Oxford University Press, 2007.

Sutherland, Olga, Andrea V. Breen, and Stephen P. Lewis. "Discursive Narrative Analysis: A study of Online Autobiographical Accounts of Self-Injury." *Qualitative Report* 18, no. 48 (2013): 1–17.

Suyemoto, Karen L. "The Functions of Self-Mutilation." *Clinical Psychology Review* 18, no. 5 (1998): 531–554. doi:10.1016/S0272-7358(97)00105-0

Tatnell, Ruth, Lauren Kelada, Penelope Hasking, and Graham Martin. "Longitudinal Analysis of Adolescent NSSI: The Role of Intrapersonal and Interpersonal Factors." *Journal of Abnormal Child Psychology* 42, no. 6 (2014): 885–896. doi:10.1007/s10802-013-9837-6

Trujillo, Natasha P., and Heather Servaty-Seib. "Parental Absence and Non-Suicidal Self-Injury: Social Support, Social Constraints and Sense-Making." *Journal of Child and Family Studies* 27, no. 5 (2017): 1449–1459. doi:10.1007/s10826-017-0976-1

Turner, Brianna J., Alexander L. Chapman, and Brianne K. Layden. "Intrapersonal and Interpersonal Functions of Non-Suicidal Self-Injury: Associations with Emotional and Social Functioning." *Suicide and Life-Threatening Behavior* 42, no. 1 (2012): 36–55. doi:10.1111/j.1943-278X.2011.00069.x

Turner, Brianna J., Matthew A. Wakefield, Kim L. Gratz, and Alexander L. Chapman. "Characterizing Interpersonal Difficulties Among Young Adults Who Engage in Nonsuicidal Self-Injury Using a Daily Diary." *Behavior Therapy* 48, no. 3 (2017): 366–379. doi:10.1016/j.beth.2016.07.001

Turner, Brianna J., Rebecca J. Cobb, Kim L. Gratz, and Alexaner L. Chapman. "The Role of Interpersonal Conflict and Perceived Social Support in Nonsuicidal Self-Injury in Daily Life." *Journal of Abnormal Psychology* 125, no. 4 (2016): 588–598. doi:10.1037/abn0000141

Vansteelandt, Kristof, Marliez Houben, Laurence Claes, Ann Berens, Ellen Sleuwaegen, Pascal Sienaert, and Peter Kuppens. "The Affect Stabilization Function of Nonsuicidal Self Injury in Borderline Personality Disorder: An Ecological Momentary Assessment Study." *Behavior Research and Therapy* 92 (2017): 41–50. doi:10.1016/j.brat.2017.02.003

Victor, Sarah E., Alison E. Hipwell, Stephanie D. Stepp, and Lori N. Scott. "Parent and Peer Relationships as Longitudinal Predictors of Adolescent Non-Suicidal Self-Injury Onset." *Child and Adolescent Psychiatry and Mental Health* 12, no. 1 (2019). doi:10.1186/s13034-018-0261-0

Walsh, Barent W., and Paul Rosen. "Self-Mutilation and Contagion: An Empirical Test." *The American Journal of Psychiatry* 142, no. 1 (1985): 119–120.

Walsh, Barent W., and Paul M. Rosen. *Self-Mutilation: Theory, Research, and Treatment*. New York, NY: Guilford Press, 1988.

Whitlock, Janis, John Eckenrod, and Daniel Silverman. "Self-Injurious Behaviors in a College Population." *Pediatrics* 117, no. 6 (2006): 1939–1948. doi:10.1542/peds.2005-2543

Wilcox, H. C., A. M. Arria, K. M. Caldeira, K. B. Vincent, G. M. Pinchevsky, and K. E. O'Grady. "Longitudinal Predictors of Past-Year Non-Suicidal Self-Injury and Motives Among College Students." *Psychological Medicine* 42, no. 4 (2012): 717–726. doi:10.1017/S0033291711001814

Wilhelm, Frank H., Paul Grossman, and Maren I. Müller. "Bridging the Gap Between the Laboratory and the Real World: Integrative Ambulatory Psychophysiology." In *Handbook of Research Methods for Studying Daily Life*, edited by Matthias R. Mehl and Tamlin S. Conner, 210–234. New York: Guilford Press, 2012.

Wilhelm, Peter, and Dominik Schoebi. "Assessing Mood in Daily Life: Structural Validity, Sensitivity to Change, and Reliability of a Short-Scale to Measure Three Basic Dimensions of Mood." *European Journal of Psychological Assessment* 23, no. 4 (2007): 258–267. doi:10.1027/1015-5759.23.4.258

Yates, Tuppett M. "The Developmental Psychopathology of Self-Injurious Behavior: Compensatory Regulation in Posttraumatic Adaptation." *Clinical Psychology Review* 24, no. 1 (2004): 35–74. doi:10.1016/j.cpr.2003.10.001

You, Jianing, Freedom Leung, and Kei Fu. "Exploring the Reciprocal Relations Between Nonsuicidal Self-Injury, Negative Emotions and Relationship Problems in Chinese Adolescents: A Longitudinal Cross-Lag Study." *Journal of Abnormal Child Psychology* 40, no. 5 (2012): 829–836. doi:10.1007/s10802-011-9597-0

Young, Robert, Nina Sproeber, Rebecca C. Groschwitz, Marthae Preiss, and Paul L. Plener. "Why Alternative Teenagers Self-Harm: Exploring the Link Between Non-Suicidal Self-Injury, Attempted Suicide and Adolescent Identity." *BMC Psychiatry* 14, no. 1 (2014). doi:10.1186/1471-244X-14-137

Chapter 6

Discursive Tensions and Contradictions

A Cultural Analysis of an Online Self-Harm Forum[1]

Mike Alvarez

MENTAL HEALTH AND SELF-HARM IN ONLINE CONTEXTS

The anonymity of online communication, and its capacity to collapse space and time, has made possible forms of sociality that were nonexistent or rare prior to the advent and commodification of the Internet. This is especially the case for individuals who in Goffman's (1963) terms carry a discredited or discreditable stigma, whose identities are marked in some way, whether or not those marks are physically apparent on the body. Such individuals include, but are not limited to, sexual minorities, the disabled, individuals with rare diseases, the terminally ill, and the mentally ill. Given that individuals with mental health conditions are several times more likely to use online support groups than people with other conditions (Owen et al. 2010), their activities online are of special concern to communication scholars.

The benefits of participating in online support groups for people with mental health concerns have been documented extensively. For instance, Baker and Fortune (2008) identify three recurring benefits among users of websites dedicated to the discussion of suicide: empathetic understanding, acquisition of coping strategies, and a sense of community. Westerlund (2013) would concur, adding that participation in such sites can sway users away from death and toward life, allowing them to renegotiate their future in dialogue with others and supplant their feelings of abnormality with that of shared humanity. Similar observations have been made by Eichhorn (2008) and by Yeshua-Katz and Martins (2013) with respect to the online activities of young women with eating disorders. Through blogs, forums, instant messaging, and other platforms of online communication, participants can offer and solicit emotional, informational, and instrumental support, express their innermost thoughts without fear of judgment or reprisal, achieve cathartic ventilation, cope with stigma, and transform weak ties between strangers into strong ties between intimates. To this list, Thompson (2012) would add, based on his study of seventeen disorder communities online, the opportunity to narrativize thoughts, feelings, and behaviors that are otherwise taboo offline, to find others who share one's stigma, to challenge unfair and disabling representations in the culture at large, and to disseminate alternative perspectives on mental health.

For every narrative about the Internet's emancipatory potential, however, there is a corresponding narrative about its potential risks and harms (Katz and Rice 2002). In the realm of mental health, such harms have also been extensively catalogued. For instance, Haas et al. (2010) speak of websites with explicitly harmful content and an anti-recovery stance, for which they have coined the term "online negative enabling support groups," or ONESG (51–52). Within such contexts, worrisome behaviors are celebrated or glorified, tips and tricks for initiating and maintaining dangerous behaviors are shared, and negative self-evaluations and self-criticisms stand uncorrected. Such groups also discursively construct non-members, including mental health professionals, as distrustful, thus deferring the possibility of help-seeking. Because one is exposed to others who share the same views, the result is a deepening of those views—a phenomenon that Baym (2010) refers to as "monadic clusters" (96). Though the concept of ONESG was derived from work with eating disorder populations, the concept has broad applicability; for instance, it can be observed in suicide-related websites that encourage suicide plans and frame death as emancipatory (Westerlund 2011, 2013) and in online contexts where participants carry out a harmful behavior so as not to lose face, often with disastrous consequences (Baum et al. 1997; Stamenkovic 2012).

Of course, even pro-recovery sites with benevolent intentions cannot guarantee the physical and psychological safety of its participants. As Yeshua-Katz and Martins (2013) point out, profound misunderstandings can arise due to the absence of non-verbal leakage cues (such as facial expressions) one ordinarily finds in face-to-face communication; a message intended to be helpful might instead be perceived as hurtful. The stakes are especially high when the recipient is in a fragile emotional state. Furthermore, the sensitivity of information disclosed online and the ease with which such information can be disseminated can also raise concerns about privacy among users.

Despite the attention funneled toward the online activities of various disorder communities and the potential benefits and harms such activities confer, the online practices of people who self-harm have been relatively understudied, especially by scholars who employ methods grounded in communication theory. In an early study, Rodham et al. (2007) conducted an interpretative phenomenological analysis of messages in a non-professional self-harm message board. Their findings reveal three recurring functions: (1) seeking validation of one's worth and confirmation of one's self as legitimate to others, (2) solicitation of support in the midst of a crisis—specifically, when the user is about to or has just engaged in deliberate self-harm, and (3) expression and cathartic ventilation of intense feelings and emotions.

Consistent with the aforementioned studies, there is a sense among users that the message board is a safe environment where they can communicate openly about subjects that are off-limits offline. Newcomers, in particular, feel welcomed by veteran users who provide an introduction to the traditions and etiquette of the board.

But while respondents are supportive and reassuring, and though self-harm is not explicitly encouraged, Rodham et al. (2007) are concerned that by sometimes framing self-harm as a "slip up," the behavior can be normalized as an acceptable method of coping with stressful circumstances; its seriousness might, therefore, be minimized. The authors also find it troubling that users do not always provide one another with alternatives to self-harm.

Smithson et al. (2011) employ discourse analytic strategies to study communication on *SharpTalk*, an online support forum for "young people who self-harm" (YPSH). Results reveal that *SharpTalk* users seek advice on practical problems in order to subsequently request emotional aid, suggesting that empathy is what is truly sought. When there is a mismatch between the expectations of posters and respondents, or when posts are unspecific (both of which can lead to "frozen threads"), respondents resort to generic displays of empathy and solidarity. Giving *and* seeking advice or support is a joint activity and responsibility assumed by users; everyone is expected to provide responses, not just to ask. Lastly, users draw on normative discourses of safety and care when giving advice to one another (e.g., proper treatment of cuts and minimization of bodily injury), which runs counter to the concern expressed by Rodham et al. (2007) that self-harm forums might encourage self-harm behavior.

A second study on *SharpTalk* (Sharkey et al. 2012) applies Goffman's (1967) concept of "face"—that is, the social self individuals present in everyday life—to explore how users' protective orientation toward one another manifest in their language use. Analyses of talk revealed attempts to reduce the likelihood of negative face threats and maintain positive face for both advice seeker and giver. These are accomplished via a number of mitigating devices. For instance, via disclaimers, users acknowledge that their advice might not be terribly useful; in doing so, they avoid issuing direct commands and save their own face should their advice be rejected or ignored. Via hedge phrases (e.g., "maybe," "perhaps") and tag questions (suggestions presented as questions), in lieu of direct advice, users also remove the "compulsion to act, from an already stressed out person" (77) and assign authority to the addressee on whom the decision to act on advice falls. Taken together, these linguistic strategies evidence *SharpTalk* users' respect for one another's autonomy and recognition of their shared vulnerability.

The brief summary of the scholarship I have provided so far illustrates that much research on online mental health communities—and online self-harm communities, specifically—focuses on cataloguing benefits and harms. This is unsurprising given that the mental health disciplines, from which such research originates, are concerned first and foremost with the identification of risk and protective factors, as well as beneficial and harmful content, contexts, and uses. But as Harvey and Brown (2012) point out, "any interventions focusing entirely on correcting behavior in [individuals] who self-harm may be incomplete or misdirected" (331); scholars must also attend to "[t]he way people formulate their accounts, deploy vocabularies and concepts, and create meaning in their particular native language" (ibid.)—in other words, to what discursive practices mean to the people who engage in them, in their own terms. The present chapter is a modest attempt to do just that: to study the online communicative practices of people who self-harm, and in turn, the systems of meaning that they discursively co-create outside of therapeutic contexts.

CULTURAL DISCOURSE THEORY AND ANALYSIS

The present chapter heeds Hecht's (2010) call to extend *culture* to entities not previously considered as such—by viewing "self-injury" as a cultural rather than a diagnostic category, and people who engage in self-injury s as members of a *speech community*, defined as a group of people who share discursive practices and expressive activities that underlie shared values, beliefs, and strategies of meaning making. "Culture" is thus defined here as an expressive system of symbols and symbolic forms that are deeply meaningful to people in place, and are historically transmitted by its members across time (Carbaugh 2012).

Specifically, I enlist cultural discourse analysis (CuDA) (Carbaugh 2007, 2017; Carbaugh and Hastings 1992; Scollo 2011) because it is a rich and powerful tool for theorizing about communication generally (and communicative practices, specifically), for describing expressive activities in great depth, and for interpreting the meaning of those activities in participants' own terms. It has a rich theoretical lineage, including the ethnography of communication framework (Hymes 1972), which sees communication as locally shaped, and theories of speech codes and cultural communication (Philipsen 1987, 1997) which see "membering" as the communal function of social interaction. CuDA also honors Geertz's (1973) commitment to thick "description," that is, understanding local customs and practices from the perspective of those who engage with them.

A key assumption of CuDA, as explicated by Carbaugh et al. (1997), is that communication is used, valued, and conceived of in locally distinctive ways ("axiom of particularity" [3–4]). It is particular to specific places, and varies from one context to the next. Furthermore, in any given place a system of communicative practices already exists, and through those practices, members of a community are able to give form, order, and meaning to their social lives ("axiom of actuality" [4]). These practices are imbued with deeply meaningful messages called "cultural discourses" [168–169]) so that when participants speak, they are not only saying something about the topic at hand, they are also making metacultural commentaries about how to act, how to feel, how to relate to others, how to be, and how to inhabit the world. Carbaugh (2007) calls these the five "radiants of meaning" (174)—acting, feeling, relating, being, and dwelling, respectively (more on these ahead)—and they are invoked every time "discursive hubs" (ibid.) are used. Discursive hubs are those words, phrases, gestures, symbols, and symbolic forms that are deeply felt and pregnant with meaning to a group, (sub)culture, or community, evidenced by their frequency of use, emphatic usage, mutual intelligibility, and accessibility to participants.

A single hub can invoke multiple radiants at once, and hubs can work singly or jointly to invoke meaning. Hubs (the explicit units) and radiants (the implicit meanings) are inseparable. Not all hubs/radiants are salient or relevant in every communicative scene, and the activation of one can activate several others. To provide one example, Alvarez (see Flanigan and Alvarez 2018) tracked the usage of "suicide" (a discursive hub of action) in an online suicide forum and discovered participant meanings about what it means to *be* "suicidal" (radiant of *being*) and *feel* "suicidal" (radiant of *feeling*), and what spatial (e.g., placelessness, entrapment) and relational (e.g., rupture, loss) conditions (radiants of *dwelling* and *relating*, respectively) precipitate suicidality.

The relationship between hubs and radiants can perhaps be more clearly understood by picturing a wagon wheel. Imagine that the circumference of this wheel has five spokes; these correspond to the five types of discursive hubs. When following the hub from the surface to the center, one realizes that this center connects to all the other hubs. That is because this center is the expressive system of meanings from which all other meanings radiate.

For my research method in this chapter, I analyzed a sample of 223 messages posted by seventy-nine anonymous users in a single online thread in which participants discuss their reasons for self-harming. The thread, whose messages were posted over a period of fourteen months, can be found in SuicideForum.com, one of the largest websites dedicated to the discussion of suicide and self-harm, with over 120,000 threads, 1.4 million replies, and 27,000 members from across the globe. Started in 2005, SF (as its members call it), is a "peer to peer community support forum and chatroom for people in need" (www.suicideforum.com/about-sf/). It abides by a "Do no harm, promote no harm principle": While participants are free to discuss their history of suicide and/or self-injury, they are prohibited from discussing or encouraging specific plans that would endanger themselves and/or others. This rule is enforced by moderators who redact messages with content deemed to be triggering. In addition to the forums, the site provides reference materials on various mental health issues and numbers for crisis hotlines and links to crisis websites for seventy-nine countries. Formal membership is not required to access most of the site's content, but in order to post messages and participate in conversations, visitors must become registered members. Membership is free and requires no name or other personally identifying information. Communication in SF is primarily in English.

Analytically, I treat SuicideForum.com as the *communication scene* in question, defined by Hymes (1972) as the setting or place in which communication occurs. The specific thread under study is treated here as a *communication event*, a sequence of purposeful communicative acts that follow a logical sequence and flow (Hymes 1972). For the purposes of this study, the communication event's beginning is defined as the thread's first post (by the topic creator, or TC), with the end corresponding to the thread's final post.

It must be noted that not all members of SF engage in self-injurious behavior, but all members who participated in the thread claim to. Furthermore, not all self-harming members of SF are actively suicidal, though many certainly are. Thus, it might be more accurate to treat SF members, writ large, as members of a cultural category, and self-harming participants as members of a unit within that larger category.

I focused on a single discursive hub—"self harm" (a hub of action)—systematically tracking participants' usage of the term (and its variants, like "self-injury" or "SH") in order to arrive at corresponding radiants of meaning. As mentioned, because a single hub can activate multiple radiants at once, I posited one research question for each radiant of meaning, as follows:

1. Acting: What models for social action are presumed when self-harm is enacted?

2. Feeling: What models for the expression and regulation of emotion are presumed when self-harm is enacted?
3. Relating: What is presumed about social relationships when self-harm is enacted?
4. Being: What models of personhood are presumed when self-harm is enacted?
5. Dwelling: What is presumed about place when self-harm is enacted?

I present interpretive accounts in the form of *cultural premises* (italicized throughout), defined by Carbaugh (2007, 2017) as abstract formulations that capture participants' taken-for-granted knowledge and beliefs about the current state of things ("what is") and evaluative judgments about the ideal state of things ("what ought to be"). Each cultural premise is supported by brief excerpts from the forum thread. As mentioned earlier, not all radiants are relevant in every communicative scene, and because the radiant of *dwelling* was not invoked in participants' online discourse, the fifth research question could not be answered satisfactorily.

Before I present findings, a few words on ethics are in order. The analysis of messages on SuicideForum.com was based on extant data online; neither intervention nor interaction with users actually took place. Analysis was limited only to publicly accessible forums with heavy traffic, and the comments are not linked to individually identifiable information such as real names, dates of birth, e-mail addresses, and social security numbers, only to usernames and avatars. Of course, Internet users sometimes use their actual names as their username and their photographs in real life as their avatar, but this did not appear to be the case for the thread I analyzed. Nonetheless, I followed the ethical guidelines set forth by the Association of Internet Researchers (Markham and Buchanan 2012) throughout my analysis.

A related concern raised by Stern (2003) pertains to the ethical and legal responsibilities of researchers upon encountering distressing information, such as users threatening to inflict bodily harm upon themselves. However, because SF prohibits users from sharing suicide plans and self-harm methods, and because posts containing triggering information are promptly deleted by moderators, I did not encounter posts that warranted intervention within the "pro-life" (users' words, not mine) context of SF.

MEANINGS ACTIVATED IN SELF-HARM DISCOURSE

In what follows, I explore emotional precipitants to self-harm that are active in users' online communication, including the "urge" that drives the act, after which I explicate the myriad ways self-injurious behavior manages intense experiences and emotions. Then, I situate the act within discourses about relationships, tracking both relational precursors to self-harm and the relational purposes for which self-harm is enlisted. Lastly, I excavate notions of personhood, and the value or worth attached to self, embedded in forum participants' discourse.

Emotional Precipitants to Self-Harm

It is apparent from the discourse of participants who self-injure on SuicideForum.com that their *self-harm behaviors are precipitated by intense emotions which the self-injurious behavior is used to manage*. These emotions encompass a wide gamut including sadness, anger, panic, anxiety, despair, and regret. For instance, one participant attributes their most recent attempt at self-harm to "panicking about the weekend's family dinner" which has been a source of undue stress for this individual.

The management of emotion via self-injury is not so straightforward, however. *One affective state can trigger other affective states before the need to self-injure arises*, and depending on the person, *some feelings are more closely associated with self-injury than others*. These two points are apparent in the following forum post: "Whenever i get sad, i get angry. whenever i get angry i . . . ." For this user, anger is the precipitant to self-injury, but sadness here is also linked to self-injury, albeit indirectly.

Interestingly, positive feelings can also act as precipitants: "I'm mostly happy and had a good day. But all of a sudden I started wanting to hurt myself." This is linked to *notions of the self as "inadequate" and undeserving of happiness* (I return to this point later), such that joy is perceived as unreal when actually experienced, as one participant's comment shows: "I'm in a good place at the moment (I wouldn't say happy but it's the closest thing I've been in a long time) and this morning I woke up with the urge to SH. Maybe it's a 'I can't believe I'm feeling good pinch me and I'll wake up' kinda thing." Joy here is framed as surreal, outside the realm of the writer's day-to-day experience, so that when it is felt, it is not expected to last.

Perhaps it would be more accurate to say that the feeling immediately precipitating self-injurious behavior is the very "need" to self-harm, which users discursively co-construct as a "compulsion" or "urge." "The urge to self harm can be very powerful," writes one SF user. Such an urge is so powerful, it is visceral, which another user describes as "This tense feeling in my stomach that feels like I won't be satisfied until I'm bleeding." When the urge surfaces it is seemingly insurmountable: "No amount of running, counting to 10, etc. can stop the urge when it surfaces," "I feel like there is only one way to stop it and that's to just get it over with."

The urge is so strong it seems to take a life of its own; in fact, it is sometimes personified in self-injury discourse: "I cut because the little voice in my head said I could, I would and I should so I did." As this metaphorical example illustrates, the compulsion to self-harm appears to possess such agency that one has no choice but to succumb to its demands.

The compulsion to self-harm grows over time ("The feeling to do so had grown. Day by day. Hour by hour. Minute by minute"), but while it is a constant presence in the lives of individuals, the urge waxes and wanes, punctuated by moments of reprieve. This is evident in the following messages, which enlist the metaphor of a crisis that will eventually pass: "Please call a crisis hotline so you can get the support you deserve *until the storm passes* and you find your own strength again," "I hope this'll *pass*," and "let these thoughts *ride out*" (italics added for emphasis).

It is important to note that forum participants do share non-injurious alternatives to self-harm. These include running ice cubes along one's arm, using an elastic band on one's wrist, writing with a red marker on one's arm to simulate blood, splashing cold water on one's face, listening to music, calling a helpline, phoning a friend, guided meditation, physical exercise, and writing one's thoughts, just to name a few. In fact, the *urge or compulsion to self-harm is something that must be actively resisted* ("I will try to keep from hurting myself"), a premise that is underscored by the following adversarial phrases: "I'm going to *work against* it though," "I'm doing my best to *fight back*," and "I have been *fighting* the urge to SH for a bit now" (italics added). Members are quick to offer words of encouragement to those who struggle to abstain from self-injury: "I hope you don't give in" and "Hang in there hun!" These self-harm alternatives are themselves discursive hubs of action whose invocation in discourse suggests that self-harm is a less preferred method for stress and emotion management.

Of course, resisting the urge can often feel like "a losing battle," especially when the "relief [self-injury] brings" is immediate (albeit temporary). For several users, *resisting takes so much effort and deliberation*—as opposed to self-injury, which has become almost reflexive and instinctual—that the urge often triumphs: "But I don't have time for this 'will-I-won't-I' type of thing that usually happens when I'm thinking of self-harming," and "Thinking of just cutting myself to get it over with so I don't waste any more time thinking about it and I can just move on."

Self-harm, then, is enacted when alternatives are deemed inefficacious, and when no other options for the management of emotions are forthcoming, as these comments suggest: "I don't know what else to do to help atm [at the moment]," "elastic bands and ice don't work for me . . . i need to see the colour red [. . .] and drawing on my skin with a red (pen) doesn't work either," "I don't know what to think about my elevated levels of anger and resentment [. . .] I don't know how to mitigate them, or rather, I don't perceive mitigating them any other way. Self-harm is a clear option, and an appealing one at that." Although self-harm is the less preferred method for managing emotions, it is apparent in discourse that it is a more efficacious and immediately gratifying action than non-injurious alternatives.

What makes self-harm even more difficult to resist is that *reminders of the behavior can trigger the act itself.* One forum user who is writing a novel about self-injury writes: "Describing the young woman breaking her self-harm 'sobriety' . . . it's triggering me like mad." The use of the word "sobriety" is very meaningful here, for as Harvey and Brown (2012) point out, self-harm discourse is often couched in the language of substance abuse and addiction, lending further credence to the perceived insurmountability of the urge. For other forum users, televisual representations of self-harm and the fear that the urge may surface can incite the urge: "It sounds stupid . . . but the fear that the show I'm watching tonight will trigger my PTSD and my self harm impulse that it did last week . . . that fear is making me want to self harm." *Self-harm can thus be self-perpetuating,* such that for one user, "Just seeing the words 'self harm' reminded me that I wanted to do it."

The Management of Emotion

As the examples above make clear, the primary role of self-harm in the daily lives of forum participants is the management of emotion in the face of stressful life circumstances. However, the ways through which this is accomplished by the act are highly variable. For some, *self-harm is enacted so that one may feel alive, to counteract a sense of unreality and numbness*, as the following comments illustrate:

> I self harm because it's the only thing that makes me feel alive and takes awa[y] the numb feeling I have.
> When I'm losing the sense of reality, when I don't know who I am or what I am doing here, when I feel emptiness and that feeling is about to swallow me, I cut.
> I just need to feel something. Tired of being numb all the f****** time.
> The urge to self harm, for me, stems from a way to feel something. Everything I've been through, it makes me numb [. . .] When I self harm, it's to feel something, to see that I'm still human.

For these individuals, the act of self harm is linked to an ontology of the self in which mere biological existence does not guarantee a sense of aliveness. One's being in the world, so to speak, is not a sure thing, and one is prone to suffer derealization, which must then be countered by self-injurious behavior.

The need to self harm may also arise in reaction not to a deficit of feelings, but to a surplus of feelings. In such scenarios, the person may feel as if s/he is about to explode from an accumulation of negative affect, which must then be released by cutting or inflicting injury upon oneself. The following messages capture the notion of self-harm as catharsis and pressure relief:

> I already have enough [on] my plate so something has gotta happen to relieve the pressure
> cutting will release some of this build up
> For me it's a release from all negative thoughts and feelings.
> it's a release . . . . like a dam breaking or when you finally breathe out after holding your breath for a time

The invocation of a dam and suspension of one's breath are particularly illustrative of the sense of being overwhelmed, as if one were being swept away by torrential affect, with self-harm as the only visible anchor. The enactment of self-harm can "release" (again, temporarily) not only the build-up of painful affect, but the thoughts and memories that produce such affect: "All the sad thoughts in my head about all the things that never were and should have been . . . and all the things that shouldn't have happened," "Memories of being a terrible person and having done terrible things," and "Wanting to rid my mind of abusive stuffs [sic]."

Self-harm as response to a paucity of affect, and self-harm as response to an excess of affect, are not mutually exclusive. The same individual may experience both states at different points in time and still enlist the same behavioral response, as the following user suggests when asked why s/he self-harms: "Because I need to calm down, to feel something, to obtain release." The need "to feel something" implies a deficit of affect, whereas the need "to obtain release" implies its accumulation, yet in this example they are invoked simultaneously.

Self-harm can also work via transmutation—specifically, by turning mental or emotional pain into physical pain, or by replacing the former with the latter. In self-injury discourse, there appears to be an economy of pain in which physical pain is less in magnitude than emotional pain, and, therefore, more manageable, tolerable, and preferable.

> I feel like I need to manifest the emotional pain and stress onto my body.
> In my mind, bleeding out is more of a relief [than] my depression
> The desire to replace mental pain with physical pain [is] because it's easier to bare for me.
> the pain I feel for several days until it's healed is distraction. physical pain is creating an escape from inner pain, which can't be put in words, can't be addressed.
> Wanting to feel something physical. Too tired of emotional pain.

Of course, forum participants recognize in discourse that the transmutation of emotional into physical pain is not a long-term solution, but a temporary one. Some have even described self-harm as a mere distraction: "Shifts the focus, even for a minute to what is at hand. While a temporary distraction . . . A distraction nonetheless." Others have described it as deflection or rerouting: "I have hypertension and anxiety, it re directs the pain," "Pain accumulated in one area gets to be overwhelming (mental pain); I want to cause pain elsewhere."

The enactment of self-harm can also displace violent feelings intended for others onto oneself. In other words, in lieu of causing injury to another, one injures oneself: "Wanting to relieve pressure and frustration and I don't want to hurt anyone else," "I get aggressive so easily and since I don't want to hurt others I pile it up and turn it on myself," and "[what] makes me want to hurt myself [is] anger and the feeling that I could hurt him." Thus, not only can self-harm transmute emotional pain into physical pain, it can also displace that discomfort onto other targets. This suggests that in order for there to be some relief, pain must have a target, even if the target is not the rightful recipient.

As paradoxical as it may seem, *the enactment of self-harm can serve to counteract suicidality* and, therefore, allow one to continue living. According to one participant, injuring oneself "feels better than the alternative," which is to die by one's hands. Others have expressed a similar sentiment, writing that self-harm is "how I [rid] myself of suicidal thoughts," and that it "helps me to survive everyday." It can keep suicidal thoughts in check, keeping them from "escalating," or at the very least, distract oneself and "change my mind off the subject."

The deterrent function of self-harm has been observed by Ekman and Söderberg (2008) in their study of the online activities of women diagnosed with borderline personality disorder who viewed self-harm as restitutive rather than destructive. But as Joiner (2005) cautions, the road to suicide can also be constructed by repeated attempts at bodily injury which can render oneself inured to physical pain and, eventually, to the thought that one can bring about the end to one's life. The notion of self-harm as an avenue to eventual suicide is evident in the following forum post: "Cutting and slipping away into death is all I can [think] about." And herein lies another paradox: Self-harm can serve as both protection against and precursor to suicide.

Ultimately, what is deemed truly restitutive by several participants is to let one's emotions run their "natural" course, as the following interchange suggests:

Poster: "I spent most of this weekend crying. I really hate to cry because it makes me feel weak. But to be honest the crying really helped and I eventually forgot about hurting myself."

Respondent: "[Y]ou were able to recognise your emotions and allow them to run their course without simply resorting to SH and just push them down [. . .] Sometimes we have to make ourselves vulnerable and weak in order to become stronger."

By allowing oneself to ventilate one's feelings without recourse to self-injury, genuine relief is experienced. This, of course, presents a challenge because self-harm is often perceived to be necessary in facilitating emotional expression or cathartic ventilation, and the urge or compulsion to self-harm can overwhelm attempts to abstain from or defer the act.

Self-Harm in Relational Context

The act of self-harm, and the feelings that precipitate and follow the act, are inextricably bound to other persons in the lifeworld of the person who self-injures. A common theme in the messages analyzed is *relational rupture as precipitant to self-harm*, as illustrated by the following example:

> Typically the urge to self harm comes when my husband and I are arguing, usually this argument involves a mistake I made almost a decade ago. Especially if I'm feeling particularly like I've failed, that's when hurting myself just *calms* me, sort of separates myself from the situation. It's almost always when I'm feeling like I failed as a person, in my relationship or as a mother.

In this example, the urge to self-harm, and the act itself, are preceded by marital conflict. The conflict is taken as evidence of the speaker's failure to fulfill relational roles, which in turn implicates the self and its perceived lack of worth for others. This example also challenges popular conceptions that non-suicidal self-injury (NSSI) is restricted to adolescents; here, the poster is a grown woman, a mother, and wife. Of course, relational rupture assumes many guises, such as mistreatment ("bullied by others"), abuse ("Lifelong abuse with no hope of it ever ending"), ostracism ("Being constantly ignored and feeling invisible"), social devaluation ("Not being valued or appreciated"), and manipulation ("being manipulated or used like a pawn").

Self-injury can make one's emotional pain visible to others, so that these others can apprehend the depths of one's suffering, as the following messages suggest:

> I feel like I have to do something drastic so they understand how bad things really are inside my head.
> I'm under a lot of stress and the pressure is building . . . in some strange twisted way I want people to see what they've done to me and because I can't

> articulate my feelings and how stressed and anxious I am I just want to have a physical manifestation on the outside to show how upset I am on the inside. [C]arving into my body will cue others into how much pain I am in.

The body and the scars it bears can, therefore, serve as testimony to the emotional injuries one has sustained, including those inflicted by others, and especially when words fail—a claim supported by Atwood (2012).

Self-harm can even serve as retaliation against offending others and as corrective to misimpressions: "I want to hurt him and prove I wasn't crying wolf and seeking attention." Alternately, the act can measure others' concern for the well-being of the person who self-injures: "Sometimes I want to hurt myself to test my friends and family, and see if they would observe anything, or even care." If others notice and express recognition of the injury or scar, then they "care"; if they fail to notice, then they don't care.

If self-harm can concretize emotional pain for the apprehension of others, then it may seem ironic when forum participants enact self-harm to achieve isolation: "I see scars as the way to justify my actions. 'look at me, I have scars, I bled yesterday, don't expect me to be normal, *leave me alone*'" (italics added). The picture is further complicated when one considers that a pervasive sense of isolation can incite self-harm: "My triggers normally arise *when there's nobody I can talk to* and so I keep all my emotions to myself, they fester until the point I want a physical release" and "sometimes I can't [breathe] through the tide of loneliness and loss" (italics added). In short, *self-harm can lead to isolation and isolation can lead to self-harm, yet in the language of self-harm, a yearning for recognition is embedded*.

So far, I have positioned the act of self-harm within relational contexts that can be described as negative. Common sense would suggest that *positive relationships can mitigate or attenuate the need to self-harm*, and there is certainly evidence of this in forum participants' discourse. Positive relationships can take the form of a support system, and they can be formal ("DBT [dialectical behavior therapy] is a huge step forward") or informal ("a friend helped boost my confidence").

Some words of caution are in order, however. Formal support is not always viewed favorably by participants, especially when the professional accuses the person who engages in self-injury of "attention seeking," as one exasperated user laments: "So fed up of professionals telling me my point of view means shit and just treating me as such." For an encounter to be therapeutic or restorative, one's point of view must be taken as valid. Furthermore, even when support systems are deemed beneficial, participants may feel guilty for the care that they receive: "Sometimes I almost hate how much my friends love me. I feel like they hurt because of it and it's all my fault." This is because participants feel undeserving of support, which is tied to a view of the self as lacking in worth, to which I now turn.

Self-Harm and Self-Worth

Forum participants discursively construct *the self as lacking intrinsic value or worth*. "I'm a worthless piece of shit," posted one user. "I don't matter and am pathetic and shouldn't exist," posted another. "Fuck my fucking idiotic existence." But the self is not only valueless, it is lacking in value for others, as these comments show: "I am [a] huge disappointment and a waste of space," "Feeling numb, nothing, like I don't matter, that I will never be taken seriously," and "The fact that I will never be good enough to be loved makes me want to hurt myself." Trapped in a vicious cycle, these individuals "self harm when [they] feel useless," with the act itself serving as confirmation that they are indeed "weak" or "useless," for they have succumbed to the urge to self-harm.

A corollary to the notion of self as valueless is the notion that *one is also a failure*. The smallest hint of failure in meeting the demands of daily life can incite self-harm. Though these precipitants might appear trivial to others, they are treated as valid sources of distress by forum participants, taken as evidence that one is truly defective or lacking: "Whenever I feel like I've failed, whether it's not doing my homework or not responding to texts," "Anything that distresses me. From having bad grades . . . to a simple comment" and "I just bombed my political science test."

Failure that is projected into the future can also incite self-harm. This is exemplified by the user who "bombed" his/her political science exam and who writes in a subsequent post: "I probably won't be able to afford to take the GRE for admission into grad school and might not even be able to afford application fees for grad school so I'll never achieve my dreams." In short, whether real or imagined, located in the past or projected into the future, *failure is magnified and taken as evidence of a defective self*.

If one is a failure, then one is deserving of pain and punishment: "I deserve to hurt," "I need [to] punish myself for not being good enough," "I feel like I'm doing myself a favour by suffering," and "[pain] helps me feel like I am getting what I deserve." But even when pain and punishment (in the form of self-injury) are received, they are simply not enough ("I deserve far worse"); they must be increased in quantity by oneself or by others ("I feel that people are going too easy on me or I haven't been punished enough"). Any less is incommensurate with one's inherent sense of worthlessness.

It is not surprising that when participants speak of misfortune, they say that they "deserve" it, but when the conversation turns to good fortune, they say that they are undeserving ("I don't deserve to be happy"). This orientation to life can make it difficult for participants to "let myself enjoy [the] day." It may also lead participants to question their continuing aliveness: "Just the fact that I'm alive, that I haven't killed myself makes me feel like I need to self harm because I'm a coward for still being here." Previously, I noted that self-harm can be a means of *staying* alive, but here it is enacted as punishment for *being* alive.

It is not only the self that must be punished, but the uncooperative body as well. In a strange twist of irony, physical pain that arises spontaneously, such as headaches and knee pains, or a stomach that grumbles when one does not feel like eating, is grounds for self-injury. But as participants' comments suggest, like the transmutation of physical into emotional pain via self-injury, *enacting self-harm to override spontaneous bodily pain is a form of mastery*, of exercising power by disciplining the body and mind: "By cutting, I feel like I'm in control" and "I want to be in control of at least some of my pain, even if it's pain I give myself." Implicit in this proposition is a view of the self as being utterly powerless. But if the self is powerless and self-harm grants a modicum of control, then this control is effectively nullified by one's powerlessness in the face of the urge to self-harm.

CULTURAL PREMISES REVISITED

To bring this chapter to a close, I summarize the cultural propositions, or taken-for-granted cultural knowledge and beliefs, that are active in forum participants' discourse—this time categorized by radiant. As mentioned, a single discursive hub (e.g., "self-harm") can tap into multiple radiants at once. In other words, because radiants of meaning emanate from the same nucleus—or core system of meaning—there are inevitably going to be crossovers between cultural premises, but they are formulated as such that the radiant in question is centered. For instance, the enactment of self-harm for the purpose of transmuting painful affect activates both radiants of *acting* and *feeling*, so there are going to be cultural premises on self-harm as action and on the transmutability of emotion. Again, because the radiant of *dwelling* was not meaningfully invoked in the messages analyzed, no cultural propositions for this radiant are offered. As these propositions further illustrate, the online discourse of self-injury is indeed rife with tensions and contradictions.

Acting

At its core, self-harm is a form of self-mastery. It can discipline the uncooperative body and manage intense feelings temporarily. The act is preceded by an urge that one must actively resist. Thus, it is enacted when non-injurious alternatives are ineffective and when no other options are foreseeable. But self-harm is self-perpetuating, and reminders of the behavior can be triggering. If one can defer self-harm despite the overwhelming urge, other opportunities for emotion management may open up (e.g., crying), and these may result in genuine relief.

Functionally, self-harm can counteract a lack of feeling by helping one to feel alive. It can also counteract a surplus of feelings by releasing a build-up of emotions. Additionally, self-harm can purge thoughts and memories that cause negative feelings, turn mental or emotional pain into physical pain (which is preferable), and redirect pain intended for one target onto another (the self). Paradoxically, self-harm can keep one alive by counteracting thoughts and feelings of suicide, but it can also be punishment for being alive, and through habituation, encourage suicidal behavior in the future.

Feeling

The online discourse of people who self-injure presumes that intense feelings, both positive and negative, can be managed by self-harm. Some feelings are more closely associated with self-harm than others; the feelings in question varies from person to person. The compulsion or urge to self-harm is itself a feeling, a very powerful one that waxes and wanes, but continually grows over time. It is a feeling that must be actively resisted, however challenging.

A person can oscillate between feeling too much and too little, between feeling alive and unalive, and both affective extremes can be corrected by self-harm. According to self-injury discourse, emotional pain is in many ways mutable by self-harm. Its build-up can be released and the attendant bad thoughts and memories purged. Emotional pain can also be rerouted from one target to another or transmuted into physical pain, which is far more bearable, and hence, preferable.

The feeling of relief that results from self-harm is temporary. Genuine and lasting relief is only possible when one allows painful feelings to flow without resorting to self-harm—for instance, verbalizing stories and their attendant emotions with an empathetic and nonjudgmental listener. However, the urge can overwhelm any attempts at abstinence.

Relating

One set of cultural premises speaks to the social uses of self-harm. Relationally, self-harm can communicate the depth of one's suffering to others by making emotional pain visible on the body. It can also be a means of gauging others' concern for one's well-being and soliciting recognition and care. Conversely, self-harm can serve as retaliation against offending parties, correct others' misimpressions (e.g., that one is crying wolf), and help one achieve momentary isolation by pushing people away.

Another set of cultural premises speaks to the relational antecedents of self-harm. Ruptures in social relationships can incite self-harm, as could one's failure to fulfill social obligations; both call into question one's social worth (or lack thereof). It is important that one's humanity is recognized by others because when the validity of one's point of view is respected, a meaningful (and perhaps therapeutic) encounter may result.

Being

People who engage in self-injury often feel powerless, and through self-harm, they can achieve temporary power—for instance, by disciplining the uncooperative (and emotionally numb) body, whose scars can attest to emotional injuries suffered. But the sense of mastery provided by self-harm eventually loses effect, at which point, the sense of powerlessness further deepens.

The person who self-injures presumes him/herself to be inadequate, undeserving of happiness, and deserving of only pain and punishment. S/he is lacking in value or social worth, a failure in many senses of the word. Although the person who self-injures sometimes wishes to be left alone, s/he ultimately yearns to be taken seriously and to be recognized or understood by others.

CONCLUDING REMARKS

The discursive practices of individuals who engage in NSSI—and the meanings they discursively co-create—can be quite elusive given the social stigma of mental illness and self-harm. However, the temporal and spatial affordances of computer-mediated communication have enabled the formation of online mental health communities, making the online practices of people who self-injure visible and ripe for ethnographic inquiry. As this chapter illustrates, CuDA (Carbaugh 2007) can be a powerful tool for understanding what self-harm, as a communicative act, means to those who engage in it. It does so by attending to self-harm systemically, to the meanings about human action, emotion, social relationships, and personhood that are active in self-injury discourse.

The present study is a modest one in that it is limited to communication in a single online thread, one that is specifically about why users engage in NSSI. Future research can attend to communication across multiple threads and websites to test the external validity or generalizability of the cultural premises identified here. Given the relatively small sample of messages I analyzed, non-trivial hubs pertaining to dwelling were absent from the data; a larger corpus of data will no doubt reveal cultural premises about place.

Although the thread makes scarce mention of treatment and recovery, the study is not without implications for clinical and therapeutic practice. For instance, participants clearly understand the need to defer self-harm until pathways to more genuine and lasting relief open up. In practice, the clinician needs to introduce healthier ways of managing, rerouting, and transmuting emotional pain. Because the negative feelings that precipitate self-harm varies from person to person, strategies need to be tailored to the individual. Future research may suggest other avenues for augmenting or remediating existing paradigms of care, ideally those that take into account the lived experience and grounded perspective of people who self-injure.

NOTE

1. Abbreviations specific to this chapter: CuDA (cultural discourse analysis), ONESG (online negative enabling support groups), TC (topic creator) and YPSH (young people who self-harm).

REFERENCES

Atwood, George E. *The Abyss of Madness*. New York, NY: Routledge, 2012.
Baker, Darren, and Sara Fortune. "Understanding Self-Harm and Suicide Websites: A Qualitative Interview Study of Young Adult Website Users." *Crisis* 29, no. 3 (2008): 118–122.
Baume, Pierre, Christopher H. Cantor, and Andrew Rolfe. "Cybersuicide: The Role of Interactive Suicide Notes on the Internet." *Crisis* 18, no. 2 (1997): 73–79.
Baym, Nancy K. *Personal Connections in the Digital Age*. Malden, MA: Polity, 2010.
Carbaugh, Donal. "Cultural Discourse Analysis: Communication Practices and Intercultural Encounters." *Journal of Intercultural Communication Research* 36, no. 3 (2007): 167–182.
Carbaugh, Donal. "A Communication Theory of Culture." In *Inter/Cultural Communication: Representation and Construction of Culture*, edited by Aanastacia Kurylo, 69–87. Thousand Oaks, CA: Sage, 2012.
Carbaugh, Donal. "Terms for Talk, Take 2: Theorizing Communication Through Its Cultural Terms and Practices." In *The Handbook of Communication in Cross-Cultural Perspective*, edited by Donal Carbaugh, 15–28. New York, NY: Routledge, 2017.
Carbaugh, Donal, and Sally O. Hastings. "A Role for Communication Theory in Ethnography and Cultural Analysis." *Communication Theory* 2, no. 2 (1992): 156–165.
Carbaugh, Donal, Timothy Gibson, and Trudy Milburn. "A View of Communication and Culture: Scenes in an Ethnic Cultural Center and a Private College." In

Emerging Theories of Human Communication, edited by Branislov Kovačić, 1–24. Albany, NY: SUNY Press, 1997.

Eichhorn, Kristen Campbell. "Soliciting and Providing Social Support Over the Internet: An Investigation of Online Eating Disorder Support Groups." *Journal of Computer-Mediated Communication* 14, no. 1 (2008): 67–78.

Ekman, Inger and Stig Soderberg. "'Across the Street—Not Down the Road': Staying Alive Through Deliberate Self-Harm." In *Internet and Suicide*, edited by Leo Sher and Alexander Vilens, 221–232. Hauppauge, NY: Nova Science Publishers, 2009.

Flanigan, Jolane, and Mike Alvarez. "Cultural Discourse Analysis as Critical Analysis: A View from Twin Oaks and SuicideForum.com." In *Engaging and Transforming Global Communication Through Cultural Discourse Analysis: A Tribute to Donal Carbaugh*, edited by Michelle Scollo and Trudy Milburn, 73–90. Madison, NJ: Fairleigh Dickinson University Press, 2018.

Geertz, Clifford. *The Interpretation of Cultures: Selected Essays*. New York, NY: Basic, 1973.

Goffman, Erving. *Stigma: Notes on the Management of Spoiled Identity*. New York, NY: Simon & Schuster, 1963.

Haas, Stephen M., Meghan Irr, Nancy A. Jennings, and Lisa M. Wagner. "Communicating Thin: A Grounded Model of Online Negative Enabling Support Groups in the Pro-Anorexia Movement." *New Media & Society* 13, no. 1 (2010): 40–57.

Harvey, Kevin, and Brian Brown. "Health Communication and Psychological Distress: Exploring the Language of Self-Harm." *Canadian Modern Language Review* 68, no. 3 (2012): 316–340.

Hecht, Michael L. "The Promise of Communication in Large-Scale, Community-Based Research." In *Distinctive Qualities in Communication Research*, edited by Donal Carbaugh and Patricia M. Buzzanell, 53–72. New York, NY: Routledge, 2010.

Hymes, Dell. "Models of Interaction of Language and Social Life." In *Directions in Sociolinguistics: The Ethnography of Communication*, edited by John Gumperz and Dell Hymes, 35–71. New York, NY: Holt, Rinehart & Winston, 1972.

Joiner, Thomas. *Why People Die by Suicide*. Cambridge, MA: Harvard University Press, 2005.

Katz, James E., and Ronald E. Rice. *Social Consequences of Internet Use: Access, Involvement, and Interaction*. Cambridge, MA: MIT Press, 2002.

Markham, Annette, and Elizabeth Buchanan. *Ethical Decision-Making and Internet Research: Recommendations from the AoIR Ethics Working Committee*, 2012. Retrieved December 1, 2017, from http://www.aoir.org/reports/ethics2.pdf.

Owen, Jason E., Laura Boxley, Michael S. Goldstein, Jennifer H. Lee, Nancy Breen, and Julia H. Rowland. "Use of Health-Related Online Support Groups: Population Data from the California Health Interview Survey Complementary and Alternative Medicine Study." *Journal of Computer-Mediated Communication* 15, no. 3 (2010): 427–446.

Philipsen, Gerry. "The Prospect for Cultural Communication." In *Communication Theory: Eastern and Western Perspectives*, edited by D. Lawrence Kincaid, 245–254. Thousand Oaks, CA: Sage, 1987.

Philipsen, Gerry. "A Theory of Speech Codes." In *Developing Communication Theories*, edited by Gerry Philipsen and Terrance Albrecht, 119–156. Albany, NY: SUNY Press, 1997.

Rodham, Karen, Jeff Gavin, and Meriel Miles. "I Hear, I Listen and I Care: A Qualitative Investigation Into the Function of a Self-Harm Message Board." *Suicide & Life-Threatening Behavior* 37, no. 4 (2007): 422–430.

Scollo, Michelle. "Cultural Approaches to Discourse Analysis: A Theoretical and Methodological Conversation with Special Focus on Donal Carbaugh's Cultural Discourse Theory." *Journal of Multicultural Discourses* 6, no. 1 (2011): 1–32.

Sharkey, Siobhan, Janet Smithson, Elaine Hewis, Ray Jones, Tobit Emmens, Tamsin Ford, and Christabel Owens. "Supportive Interchanges and Face-Work as 'Protective Talk' in an Online Self-Harm Support Forum." *Communication & Medicine* 9, no. 1 (2012): 71–82.

Smithson, Janet, Siobhan Sharkey, Elaine Hewis, Ray Jones, Tobit Emmens, Tamsin Ford, and Christabel Owens. "Problem Presentation and Responses on an Online Forum for Young People Who Self-Harm." *Discourse Studies* 13, no. 4 (2011): 487–501.

Stamenkovic, Marko. "In Full View: Cybersuicide, Hypervisual Self and Public Showcase of Death (for Real)." *Medijski Dijalozi* 5, no. 12 (2012): 73–101.

Stern, Susannah R. "Encountering Distressing Information in Online Research: A Consideration of Legal and Ethical Responsibilities." *New Media & Society* 5, no. 2 (2003): 249–266.

Thompson, Riki. "Screwed Up, But Working on It: (Dis)ordering the Self Through E-Stories." *Narrative Inquiry* 22, no. 1 (2012): 86–104.

Westerlund, Michale. "The Production of Pro-Suicide Content on the Internet: A Counter-Discourse Activity." *New Media & Society* 14, no. 5 (2011): 764–780.

Westerlund, Michale. "Talking Suicide: Online Conversations About a Taboo Subject." *Nordicom Review*, no. 34 (2013): 35–46.

Yeshua-Katz, Daphna, and Nicole Martins. "Communicating Stigma: The Pro-Ana Paradox." *Health Communication* 28 (2013): 499–508.

Chapter 7

"Can Airport Scanners See Scars?"
An Interpretive Analysis of Self-Injury Narratives
Warren J. Bareiss

INTERPRETIVE INQUIRY INTO SELF-INJURY STORIES

2 months down the drain.
i was 2 months clean and then I went and fucked it up and I don't even know why
i just hate myself I feel guilty and stupid

As discussed in the previous chapter, people who self-harm can be quite eloquent in writing about their experiences, emotions, hopes, fears, and desires. The example above, featured in a Reddit forum called "r/selfharm," is a tightly packed short story bursting with palpable regret and guilt. The writer has succinctly presented deep feelings of failure to be shared with anonymous readers, many of whom will respond and contribute stories of their own. Indeed, dozens of posts appear on r/selfharm daily, illustrating the magnitude of the self-injury community.

In this chapter, I am going to operate from the perspective of an interpretive listener. By "interpretive," I mean using a scholarly frame of reference to understand symbolic codes. In this case, those codes take the form of firsthand stories about self-injury. As such, I am indebted to the work of Clifford Geertz (1973) whose *Interpretation of Cultures* has inspired generations of scholars. For Geertz, understanding cultures means using theories and concepts from anthropology, semiotics, sociology, and other relevant fields to understand the "deep structure" (p. 354) of symbolic meanings embedded in everyday words and behaviors. Understanding is always partial, however, because the interpretive frames with which we work are always limited. Interpretation is an ongoing process, not of seeking a single truth, but of recognizing that understanding is always partial and contingent on one's perspective.

Here, my "listening" pertains to the written, rather than the spoken, word. I want to "listen" carefully stories written by people who self-harm. Storytelling is a powerful tool, a means of asserting agency in the midst of adversity. Stories are a channel through which we give order to chaos and meaning to misfortune through careful framing of what happened in the past and, thus, giving reason for what is occurring right now (Riessman 1993). Stories also help people work out relationships between how they are defined by others and how they see themselves (Murray 1997). Arguably, written stories are opportunities for people who self-injure to assert *more* agency than in spoken form because writers have time to choose and arrange their words deliberately, without interruption.

In writing this chapter, I am not in the business of "giving voice" to people who engage in self-injury, nor do I claim to unlock some sort of ultimate truth about self-injury stories. As a scholar with some experience in narrative analysis, my goal is to provide my interpretation of stories, or more accurately, my interpretation of other peoples' accounts of their experiences. In no way do I want to speak *for* those who self-injure; they do a fine job of that on their own as can be seen by a cursory examination of r/selfharm and other forums. Rather, I want to look deeply into a group of stories as a way of learning about how experience is ordered and given meanings by a community of storytellers who share an intimate connection through self-injury.

Initially, I had hoped to interview students who self-injure on the campus where I teach, collecting stories about their experiences within the wider contexts of family, school, work, and so on. That plan failed due to reluctance of students to speak with me on a topic so fraught with stigma. Eventually, I discovered that social media provide contexts in which anonymity affords people who self-injure a platform to express themselves, and I found r/selfharm, to be a particularly rich source of firsthand accounts.

Reddit is a popular collection of over a million forums on all sorts of topics. Each forum is a separate "subreddit." Like all subreddits, r/selfharm is moderated by volunteers operating under guided supervision by Reddit administrators. Anyone can post to r/selfharm and respond to posts with a free account using an alias. Rules include a ban on pictures, self-harm or suicide instruction, and use of identifiable information about the sender. For this chapter, I examine fifty stories in r/selfharm posted during the summer of 2019.

As mentioned above, my approach is informed by narrative theory and research, specifically that area of narrative scholarship specializing in "illness narratives" (Frank 1998; Hyvarinen 2015; Kelly and Dickinson 1997; Riessman 2003; Seymour-Smith and Wetherell 2006), but I need to be careful to contextualize my terminology. As we have already seen in previous chapters, NSSI has been officially recognized by the American Psychiatric Association in the *Diagnostic and Statistical Manual of Mental Disorders*, fifth edition (2013). It is important to note, however, that the *DSM-V* lists NSSI as a condition for further study, rather than a specific diagnosis. Not classified as an illness in itself, NSSI is a condition indicative of other factors which could be some form of mental illness, a response to a range of life stresses with which the person has trouble coping, or a combination of both (Horner 2016; In-Albon et al. 2013; Wiseman 2018; Zetterqvist 2015).

Stories told by people struggling with illness and/or related conditions demonstrate how patients—as well as their friends and family members—perceive and engage with the world around them when intention, body, and sense of self are not quite in sync (Shimazono 2003). A pioneer in the field, Kleinman (1988) recognized that firsthand accounts told by patients can act as counter-narratives to the dominant medical model, the latter conditioned by asymmetrical doctor-patient relationships, social expectations of medical experts, and the for-profit medical industry. The medical model, Kleinman argued, often misses or ignores what illness *means* to patients, despite the fact that meaning is directly linked to awareness and appropriate action:

> Indeed, the everyday priority structure of medical training and of health care delivery with its radically materialist pursuit of the biological mechanism of disease, precludes such inquiry. It turns the gaze of the clinician, along with the attention of patients and families away from decoding the salient meanings of illness. (p. 9)

Too much focus on biological and technological factors leads to overvaluation of a generalized understanding of illness at the expense of particular, lived experience. Specific, contextual factors conditioning the individual patient's reaction to and resilience toward illness are thus at risk of being lost in the process. As noted by Frank (1995/2013), people struggling with illness, "*need* ... to tell their stories, in order to construct new maps and new perceptions of their relationships to the world" (p. 3).

Kleinman, Frank, and a little later, Charon and Montello (2002) established the foundation for what has become an extensive range of scholarship in the study of patients' stories. As Charon explained:

> Without narrative acts, the patient cannot convey to anyone else what he or she is going through. More radically and perhaps equally true, without narrative acts, the patient cannot himself or herself grasp what the events of illness mean. And without telling about or writing about the care of a patient in a complex narrative form, the caregiver might not see the patient's illness in its full, textured, emotionally powerful, consequential narrative form. It remains to be

proven—although it appears a most compelling hypothesis—that such narrative vision is required in order to offer compassionate and effective care to the sick. (Charon 2006, pp. 12–13)

Narratives provide insight into how patients (and caregivers) think—not just their perceptions of illness, but also about how they relate illness to a wide range of issues, from intensely personal and familial struggles to more general perspectives on economics, society, religion, politics, and so forth. Inquiry into stories reveals constraints and pressures faced every day that condition choices made amid limited options available. Perhaps most significant, attention paid to personal narratives is empowering to the patient, possibly leading away from feelings of helplessness toward hope and positive action.

In their analysis of interviews with people who self-injure and with their service providers, for example, Marshall and Yazdani (1999) began with the recognition that stories told about self-injury can reveal what self-harm means to those who engage in it; moreover, those stories are conditioned by other stories already circulating in the wider culture via media and interpersonal discourse. Examination of stories Marshall and Yazdani further argued, can reveal variable cultural perspectives among people who self-injure to better inform providers in understanding and serving their patients.

By interviewing people who self-injure, Chandler (2013) found that stories demonstrate a patterned form of thinking about physical pain as a form of resistance to emotional pain:

> [P]articipants described the physical pain generated by self-injury as leading to an improved sense of self.... Thus, although these narratives drew upon dualistic conceptions of self/other, mind/body, emotions/body, they simultaneously challenged the logic of these dualisms, implying a thoroughly embodied self. Thus, I would suggest that in some cases pain can be understood as reintegrating the mind/body/self rather than destroying it. This conclusion supports the argument that pain can be interpreted and experienced as productive. (p. 727)

Indeed, Chandler pushed back somewhat on narrative theorists' distrust of the medical model, noting that those who self-injure often incorporate biomedical discourse in their stories as a way to empower their own discourse and build a sense of self-efficacy.

In further research, Chandler (2014) described the narrative function of scars made by those who self-injure, arguing that scars "can be understood themselves as communicative, and narratives provided by people who are scarred provide an opportunity to control, to some extent, the nature of this communication" (p. 115). Scars, Chandler argued, provide people who self-injure starting and ending points of stories told as they want them to be told, in opposition to possible misinterpretation by others.

The participatory nature of social media makes online forums particularly valuable contexts for studying self-injury narratives (Eliseo-Arras et al. 2019; Memon et al. 2018). Inquiring into why individuals who self-injure participate in these forms of media, Seko et al. (2015) found two dominant narrative themes: *Self-oriented motivations* include reflection on what self-injury is, whereas *social motivations* pertain to seeking out and demonstrating support for others. It is worth noting that Seko, et al. found that participation in self-injury related social media both triggered *and* mitigated against further self-injury, depending upon media content and mood of the participant.

Seko and Lewis (2016) also found recurring themes in their analysis of self-injury pictures and corresponding texts posted on Tumblr. The most common recurring themes were hopefulness, hopelessness, denotation of self-injury via straightforward, descriptive imagery, and normalization—that is, presentation of self-injury "as an effective coping mechanism" (p. 190). The contradictory themes revealed by Seko and Lewis are particularly intriguing. Here, we can see how narrative analysis shows us that self-harm is far from a monolithic construct. People who self-injure approach their stories from a range of perspectives conditioned by contextual factors particular to each story and storyteller.

NARRATIVE MODEL

In the following sections, I will approach stories that people tell in r/self-harm using Frank's typology (1995/2013) consisting of three basic narrative forms: *Chaos narratives* are anti-narrative in the sense that they lack coherent structure, reflecting the contingent nature of one's existence and absence of control over one's body. *Restitution narratives* describe restoration from illness to wellness; they are often associated with the medical model wherein outside treatment is sought to restore a sense of normalcy lived prior to illness. *Quest narratives* describe transformation *through* illness; unlike restitution narratives, quest narratives are not driven by a desire to return to a pre-illness state, but rather, describe lessons in finding a new (or a more authentic) self.

Within restitution, chaos, and quest narratives, Frank notes variation among two further dimensions: body types and perceptions related to embodiment (1995/2013, p. 29). Body types consist of:

- *disciplined bodies*: emphasis on predictability and control of one's own body.
- *mirroring bodies*: based on an idealized image of a healthy body.
- *dominating bodies*: refusal to accept the contingency of one's own body leads to desire to control others.

Restitution Narrative	Chaos Narrative	Quest Narrative
• "I am sick now, but I will be well again." • Return to normalcy anticipated • Emphasis on control, return to predictability • Dissociation of self from body • Monadic perspective • Desire for return to health	• "My life is an uncontrollable mess." • Interruption of normalcy • Emphasis on lack of control, contingency • Dissociation of self from body • Monadic perspective • Lacking desire	• "You can learn from my story." • Illness as a journey toward atonement • Acceptance of contingency • Association of self and body • Dyadic perspective, communicative • Desire to help others

Figure 7.1   Frank's Three Forms of Illness Narrative. *Source*: Author created.

- *communicative bodies*: contingency is accepted as the body is used as a tool to relate to others.

Notions of embodiment comprise four continua:

- *body relatedness*: association vs. dissociation with one's body.
- *desire*: demand for more of something (e.g., time with family) vs. lack of desire.
- *other relatedness*: monadic emphasis on one's own body versus dyadic relationship with others.
- *control*: contingency vs. agency regarding one's body, in particular, and one's life more generally.

Frank's model is summarized in figure 7.1.

I am not the first to use Frank's model with respect to NSSI. Sinclair and Green (2005) and Chandler (2014) used the model to uncover recurring themes in interviews with people who had previously self-injured. Chandler points out, however, that narratives looking backward are seen through a very different lens than narratives about events in the present; as such, she invites other researchers to apply Frank's model more toward self-injury in "practice" (p. 115). This chapter accepts Chandler's invitation by examining stories told about self-injury in the present, sometimes within minutes of the event being narrated.

METHOD

I used a three-step process to analyze self-injury narratives. First, I had to determine the parameters of my sample. Using an inductive, interpretive approach, my goal was not to work toward any sort of mathematically precise sample with regard to reliability and validity. Rather, I wanted a sample that would be representative in the general sense of the word—big enough to represent types of stories present in r/selfharm, yet manageable, given the number of stories available. I began with all self-injury postings in the forum for a one-week period in the summer of 2019. Each of the messages was the first post in a thread so that responses and counterresponses are not included.

From there, I reduced the data to those messages that specifically included narratives, using Labov and Waletzky's (1967) five-part model:

- orientation: details on where and when the story took place.
- complicating action: introduction of conflict and steps taken in response to conflict.
- resolution: conclusion of the action.
- evaluation: commentary on the story including the point or moral.
- coda: what happened after the story.

Following Labov and Waletzky's admonition that all elements need not be present in each story, I included all messages that had at least four of the six narrative elements. Sorting data in this way left me with 209 stories. I then randomly selected fifty stories from the original sample: seven from each day with one extra on the last day. Once the final sample was obtained, I created a spreadsheet coding each item according to Frank's illness narrative model.

Direct quotations used in the findings below are taken verbatim from Reddit posts with original spelling and punctuation intact to preserve authors' voices. Ellipses note where I have omitted text for brevity. Also, if genders are stated in the entries, writers are referred to as "he" or "she;" otherwise, I used the gender-neutral pronoun, "they." I will use the colloquial term "Redditor" to mean anyone who posts on Reddit.

Narrative analysis sometimes uses "story" and "narrative" interchangeably. This can cause confusion when various researchers attach different meanings to each term. To be clear, throughout the remaining sections of this chapter, I will use "story" to denote accounts provided by Redditors about what happened in the past. I use "narrative" to emphasize how I categorized stories, based upon respective structural elements. *Stories* are tales told about the past, whereas *narratives* are types of stories, defined by their structure and elements.

Because Reddit is publicly available, no IRB permission was required by my university for this study. Even so, I was careful not to include any clues that might suggest a writer's identity.

OVERVIEW OF THE STORIES AND STORYTELLERS

Before moving into the narrative specifics, a few words describing the sample overall are in order. First, it is impossible to tell much about writers' identities because few provide demographic details, as per Reddit stipulations. Some details, such as mention of a school guidance counselor, reveal that many writers are adolescents; however, some contributors to r/selfharm mention having spouses and children. All posts are in English with only a few occasional clues to suggest national origin; for example, description of oneself as a "bloke" limits the story's source to the UK and a few other countries. Only one post mentions that English is not the person's native language. Based on gender cues provided, it appears that stories are written by both males and females in roughly equal proportion.

Stories in the sample are always written in the first person. The writer, in every case but one, either currently self-injures or has self-injured in the past, with the former in the majority. The one exception who has never self-injured asked for information about their sister who currently self-injures. Most often, stories described relationship problems with family members, friends, and romantic partners. Some stories are prefaced with requests for suggestions about various aspects of self-injury such as how to stop bleeding and how to hide scars.

Stories ranged from a few sentences to several hundred words. An example of a brief story is titled "Hospital:" "I'm in the ER because I cut my thigh with a razor because I'm such a basket case. I highly recommend you guys not to do this. I'll probably have to have a psych evaluation and might have to stay overnight. Fuck. I hate self-harm." Here, all the elements of Labov and Waletzky's model are concentrated within a minimum of text. The *abstract* is a one-word title revealing the general context of the story and previewing a range of possible events. The *orientation* identifies the emergency room as the specific spatial context, and the temporal context is identified as the very recent past when cutting occurred, leading to the immediate present; the reader can easily imagine a patient posting the story as they await medical attention. *Complicating action* consists of cutting with a razor blade. The narrative is only partially *resolved* with the writer ending up in the hospital, possibly overnight, awaiting a psychological evaluation (*coda*). The writer demonstrates their *evaluation* of self-injury with an expletive.

Longer stories vary in their extent of character and plot development. The longest in the sample is 850 words. The writer describes himself as a 23-year-old male who cut from the age of fourteen to sixteen, and the story describes what cutting felt like and how the writer stopped self-injuring. The story concludes with a detailed five-point list of lessons learned.

CHAOS NARRATIVES

Of the fifty stories in the sample, thirty-seven are chaos narratives. Lacking internal coherence or clear causation, these stories describe experiences of being overwhelmed in the moment. A short example is titled "After 2 months clean I've relapsed:"

> I was 2 months clean but the urges have gotten so bad lately. It felt so much easier this time too. Like I could cut as deep and as long as I wanted. And I had to make a lot more cuts then I used to before I felt satisfied. I wish I could have fought it but I feel so weak right now.

Here, the plot has to be inferred from the shreds of narrative provided. Reading the entry carefully, we can reconstruct a series of events in which the writer had self-injured up to a point two months previously. Succumbing to strong desires to resume self-injury, the writer had to do so more often than previously in order to reach the point of satisfaction. The writer regrets the self-injury and feels very weak. The type of weakness—physical, emotional, or spiritual—is unstated.

Similar chaos narratives are constructed almost like stream-of-consciousness writing, with only the thinnest of plotlines trailing off and picking up again later. One of the longer stories, for instance, recounts conflict with an unidentified authority figure:

> Haven't cut in 2-3 months. I've only had one relapse. The relapse was dealt with by threatening to take me to an autism counselor center and take away my college funding. Fine it sounds annoying and the latter petty, but eh, I'm not going to argue. Just the other day though, for whatever reason, despite not having cut/threatened to/talked about wanting to, I was straight-up fucking told for no reason other than she was thinking about my sh and scars that if I relapse, she is going to tell everyone.

That is about the first fourth of the post, the rest moving in and out of a loosely constructed narrative of how someone identified as "she" told people in the past about the self-injury, but also interspersed with reflections on the mixed value and cost of personal pride. The narrative concludes with a combination coda and evaluation:

> The reason I haven't relapsed is because of my pride. The reason I turned to self-harm in the first place? Too much pride to talk about anything. The reason I manage to roll my fatass out of bed everyday? Pride.

I guess here's to hoping shit doesn't escalate and these topics aren't brought up again in such a way. Her whole behavior about this entire situation has left me too spiteful to rationally/peacefully deal with anymore shit.

This entry evinces raw anger and frustration: anger at the threat that "she" will callously tell others about the writer's history of self-injury, and—reading between the lines—frustration at the imbalanced power relation between "she" and the writer.

Body types. Of the four body types described by Frank, by far, the most common among the chaos narratives is the communicative body. The body is a reference point—a means with which to connect with other Redditors who self-injure. Thirty-three stories—over half of the sample—fall into this category. This finding runs counter to Frank's model wherein chaos narratives are prone to monadic tendencies, "the inability to find recognition or support for the body's pain and suffering" (1995/2013, p. 102). On the other hand, this finding should not be surprising given that Reddit's purpose is explicitly *for* seeking communion with others. Another post demonstrates this function:

I just got home from a very long, hard day and ended up buying a big bag of chips and ate Everything. I got so mad at myself that suddenly I found myself standing in the bathroom, with the word "fat" cut so huge that it covers my entire stomach. Now I'm ashamed and upset with myself. I had promised myself to stop and from the looks of it, this will take a long time to heal. Mostly just needed to confess this to anyone on here/vent.

In reaching out to others, this writer rhetorically constructs a community of Redditors—what Anderson (1983) described as an "imagined community"—a rhetorical construct of imagined others with common interests who will likely never meet face-to-face.

Other relatedness. Community is further constructed via sharing and requesting advice from other imagined community members. Almost half (eighteen) of all chaos narratives in the sample exhibit dyadic relatedness to others, and an overwhelming thirty-four stories directly address the imagined audience. Both factors are in contrast to Frank's model regarding chaos narratives, again, probably due to the explicit purpose of Reddit and other social media. One writer, for example, directly addresses imagined readers about how she had cut her face and was thinking of explaining it as an accidental "shaving incident with one of those face shaving razors for girls." She closes by asking "does that sound believable?"

On the other hand, one could make the case that a monadic tendency is an important narrative feature within many stories where dysfunctional face-to-face relationships are presented, particularly regarding family relationships, for example:

> During dinner, my family were talking about self-harm and saying how they just can't understand why people cut themselves. They didn't know I self harm which is why they say all these. They were saying how people who self-harm are seeking for attention; joke about people who cut themselves are emo while saying "I cut to feel alive" in a very angsty tone. They laugh it off after, I just awkwardly laugh along. After this conversation, it made me feel so embarrassed of myself and my cuts and silently broke down in my room.
>
> I'm scared. What if they found out about my cuts one day? I don't want my family to hate or make fun of me.

This person has constructed a role to play amid the family setting, knowing that it is a fiction, and then lives in perpetual fear of being unmasked. Emotionally distanced from family, they reach out to others for understanding through r/selfharm.

Desire. For Frank, chaos narratives are marked by a lack of desire: "In a world so permeated with contingencies that turn out badly, desire is not only pointless but dangerous" (1995/2013, p. 103). This narrative dimension is the one that most differs from Frank's model among the sample stories. Indeed, nearly every chaos narrative expressed a strong desire for *something*, and this goes back to the control issue mentioned previously. What most writers in the sample want is control. Most often, writers express desire for control over their anxiety, sadness, and loneliness, with some wishing for control over their desire to self-injure:

> Throwaway. After not cutting for ten years, I cut myself yesterday. I was super drunk and actually in a really great mood and dancing and singing and then walked over to a cutting block, took out a chef knife and cut. It wasn't bad but it freaked my girlfriend out who was in the other room. I was seeing a therapist for a while but then lost my job and now don't have the money for it—anyone have any recommendations for finding better ways of coping? Going to the gym seems to help but at the same time it's just another escape. Cutting yesterday after so long of not doing it felt great and I have a huge desire to do it again but I recognize it's just a temporary escape for bigger issues that I'm not dealing with. Any recs for coping mechanisms that have worked for others would be great! Thanks!

By specifically asking for recommendations about alternative ways to cope, this person uses social media as a channel through which to attain personal agency, and thus control over their desire to self-harm. Other writers seek advice specifically about where to cut on the body, whether cuts are too deep, how scars can be hidden, and so forth—all means of expressing desire for some form of control pertaining to self-harm, contrary to Frank's model of the chaotic storyteller.

Body relatedness. Frank writes that in chaos narratives, association with the body can be hazardous: "The body is so degraded by an over-determination of disease and social mistreatment that survival depends on the self's *dissociation* from the body, even while the body's suffering determines whatever life the person can lead" (1995/2013, p. 103). Following this observation, Frank argues that in chaos narratives, storytellers tend toward dissociation. The sample examined here meets Frank about halfway, with thirteen chaos narratives leaning toward dissociation, fourteen toward association, and ten not mentioning the issue.

Dissociative perceptions are suggested in chaos narratives when writers' bodies are rhetorically constructed as something apart from the self:

> I used to not really sh, but just pinched my skin or scratched my skin off or bit the inside of my cheek. The first time actually I self harmed was kinda by accident. I was sobbing in the bathroom and my backpack kinda scratched the top of my forearm. I didn't have anything to actually cut with, so I used a sharp piece of metal from my spiral to scratch a mark onto my forearm. It took a lot of back and forth to make it bleed, but I was satisfied . . . . I made a few other feeble scratch marks around it but barely noticeable. Once I discovered razors it was a whole different story. But I still cut in the same places, there were three on top of my forearm and I used razors to make four cuts on the bottom of my forearm, like I've seen most people do. My biggest scar was from when I cut too deep on the one on top of my forearm, but I'm too embarrassed to admit that it's sh to other sh people because it just seems like such a stupid place to cut. Also I don't know many other people who just cut in the same places. I would do this to kinda "pace myself," and told myself I couldn't cut again until they healed. Of course then I got drunk and cut all over both of my arms, but nothing deep. But has anyone else cut in a place you're too embarrassed to admit because it doesn't seem like you're self harming right?

Here, the body is less equated with self-identity than as a series of places like a map, some of which are appropriate to cut, whereas others are not. Another writer similarly explains that she chooses places on her body strategically so that they will go unnoticed: "I do it on my boobs and right below my stomach cause I don't want anyone knowing . . . anyone else cut in the same spots?"

Dissociation is a controversial topic in self-injury scholarship with some scholars arguing that the lack of pain felt during self-injury episodes is evidence of dissociative episodes (see., for example, Hoyos et al. 2019). Indeed, chaos narratives in the sample not only don't mention pain, but instead, praise the positive, emotional effects of cutting.

Other researchers, however, argue that visible results of self-injury function to bring people *out of* dissociative states. Following this line of thinking, blood and scars function as visible reminders of one's physical existence (Paris 2005) in a process of reintegration (Chandler 2013). This pattern seems to be the case in a narrative mentioned above where the writer explained that "it took a lot of back and forth to make it bleed, but I was satisfied" and, in another case, an anxious mother described a calming sensation occurring after cutting and seeing blood that allowed her to fall asleep.

Another writer whose parents want to force him "back into the closet for being trans" describes in detail the frustration and anger felt at being a member of that family. The writer closes by saying, "i stopped harming and im feeling emotions again, i dont know how to cope, so how do i cope?" Again, coping and control are equated, and while this writer is starting to feel emotions without self-harm, the emotions amid their chaotic family life are upsetting. As noted above, association can be a dangerous thing in chaotic circumstances.

Rather than take a side on the dissociative/associative issue, it seems safe to conclude that storytellers in r/selfharm express both sides of the debate.

Contingency. Being at the mercy of contingent forces is the factor most in keeping with Frank's model, with thirty-three of the thirty-seven chaos narratives addressing this theme. Yet, while stories commonly lament the loss of control over external factors, many also relish in the control that self-injury provides in reducing emotional angst, as described above. The nature of self-injury helps explain this contradiction because self-injury is often a means of imposing order; the body becomes a site where the individual is in control of their pain, in contrast to the unpredictable pressures imposed from the outside world. Again, "coping" is the operative word most used in this regard:

> i'm disappointed with myself, but I know that it was the only way to cope with my anxiety in that moment. it's been 15 minutes since that now, but I feel so relaxed and peaceful. I know it shouldn't be like this, but it's very hard to quit doing it since it's an addiction I've had for more than 4 years now. does anybody else feel so calm when they self harm?

Anxiety is caused by inability to handle contingency, and cutting eases that anxiety. Note that this person characterizes cutting as a form of addiction—a common theme in the narratives. The writer faces a paradox between responding to external contingency and fueling internal compulsion in an endless round of angst, cutting, and further angst.

Less frequently, self-injury is described as self-punishment due to *lack of* control, specifically, absence of *self*-control, as in the following description:

> I cant stop hitting my self. I don't like this. I don't like how im living. I don't like who I am. I cant take it I just feel better knowing that I hit myself because im just a little bitch who deserves it.

Here, self-injury is an act of self-punishment rather than escape or relief. The same thing occurs in the post described above wherein "fat" is a pejorative label cut into the body as marker of personal weakness; the word is likely to be hidden from public view, although the story told is a confession of guilt.

So far, we have seen that chaos narratives are overwhelmingly the most common form of stories in the sample and that control (or lack of control) is a major issue. These observations should come as no surprise and are consistent with Frank's model. Less expected, however, is the fact that stories involving body types, other relatedness, desire, and body relatedness vary sharply from Frank. Some of this difference is consistent with the function of social media, whereas other variations from the model seem more akin to the specificities of NSSI, such as its secretive nature and corresponding stigma. Having discussed the most common narrative type in the sample, I now turn to narrative forms that are less common, though not less worthy of examination.

SELF-INJURY AND RESTITUTION

Restitution narratives are the second most common type of narrative present in the sample, although there are just four of these—a small fraction compared to chaos narratives. Frank describes three forms of restitution narrative: *prospective*, *retrospective*, and *institutional* (1995/2013, pp. 77–84). *Prospective* narratives project recovery at a future time ("I will be well soon"), whereas *retrospective* narratives tell about recovery that happened in the past ("I was sick and I got better"). *Institutional* narratives are most closely linked to the medical model in which an outside force, such as a pharmaceutical product or a healthcare provider, helps guide the patient toward recovery.

Of the four restitution narratives in the sample, all are either retrospective or a combination of retrospective and institutional. This pattern alone is telling in that contributors to r/selfharm tend to focus on past and current circumstances rather than on days and years to come—not surprising, given the chaotic contexts described in so many other stories.

Desire and dissociation. A cautiously optimistic desire "to get well and stay well" (Frank 1995/2013, p. 78) echoes throughout restitution narratives in the sample, for instance:

Psychiatrist had me take all the knives and razors and whatnot and put them in a hard to reach spot (they wanted me to give em to someone but i refused) so i put em in the crawlspace since its a bitch for me to get in there. They gave me meds to take as needed and for the most part its worked, i can take em when i feel the urge and it goes away, now if only the scars weren't so itchy.

Frank is suspicious of restitution narratives because they tend to reflect medical industrial sales pitches that "condition expectations" (p. 80) for how illness *is supposed to* progress, following the consumer-oriented, medical model as described earlier in this chapter. We can see a sense of that preferred perspective in this story, although it is also interesting to note that the writer does not fully comply with medical instructions by choosing to stow cutting instruments away rather than abandon them. The writer also reserves the choice whether to resume cutting or not.

The same story is consistent with Frank's assessment that restitution narratives construct the body through dissociative, mechanistic framing; however, dissociation takes a different form from what we saw in chaos narratives. Whereas chaos narratives separate self and body, restitution narratives are more likely to speak of self and scars. The writer kept the razors, and the scars are itchy reminders of their presence. As Bar-On (2014) writes,

> The scars that remain following the self-injury may arouse in the cutter a sense of existential continuity, a feeling of connection between dissociative episodes, or a sense of preserving past events or feelings that cannot be integrated into the concept of self. (p. 722)

Moving forward and away from self-injury, scars are temporal markers of past not yet relinquished.

Contingency. Unlike chaos narratives, posts describing restitution are optimistic and encouraging. Nevertheless, as with chaos narratives, contingency abounds in these accounts of restitution, where cutting is perceived to be an addiction from which one never might never fully recover:

> Hey guys! First post but I'm really excited.
>
> I've had issues with self harm for about 2 years now and it's been a month since I have self harmed. This seems small but during that month I've gone through a really rough break up, I'm home for summer in a rather stressful environment, I can't find a job, and my anxiety/depression have been bad too. Normally I'd be cutting like crazy but I've actually let myself feel my emotions. I didn't even feel the urge to cut! It's possible to move on and find other coping mechanisms.

I'm not sure I'll be clean forever but it's getting better and better. I'm seeing a therapist now too which feels good for me.

Restitution as described in this story requires drawing upon one's own agency, with the help of medical guidance, consistent with Frank's model. Nevertheless, despite steps forward, resolution is not necessarily permanent in the mind of this storyteller: "I'm not sure I'll be clean forever." Optimism is thus balanced with a darker sense of uncertainty.

The body, the self, and others. Communal discourse is unmistakable in the previous story's hail to readers ("Hey guys!"). The same story's eventual closing emphatically assures readers:

THERE IS HOPE GUYS IF I CAN DO THIS YOU CAN TOO.
anyways I love you all, stay strong
I'm always here for support too don't be shy

A better case of an imagined community would be hard to find. This writer uses their experience with cutting to model the will needed to stop self-injuring. In pledging love and offering support, the writer offers a connection that readers might not find anywhere else.

In a narrative that is remarkably similar in structure to the previous example, another writer describes short-term restitution amid recent stress:

I've been clean for a while now, a few months! But the last few days have been kind of hard and I thought about doing it. But instead I search my apartment for a rubber band to snap it agains my arm, which worked. Did it yesterday for the whole day, idk if that's bad or not. But didn't cut!

This and the previous post suggest alternatives to self-harm, thereby sharing success in overcoming self-injurious behavior—however limited and temporary that success might end up being. Contingency is accepted as a given, yet these writers assert that self-determination is still possible as they demonstrate concrete steps forward.

Another story similarly provides an alternative, safer source of physical pain, framed within communal discourse:

I have a lot of back acne and was recommended to have a bath with tea tree oil in it. I tried it and my whole body stang and burned a little. My skin was a tiny bit red afterwards but it faded quickly. I used to cut myself (right now I'm about half year clean) and this does help a little

Edit: by this post I didn't mean to say that scars are bad or anything. I have them too. But maybe if someone is in the process of being clean then you can use this tip :)

This writer is careful to balance the story of their own success with a desire not to alienate readers. The coda added at the end gently emphasizes commonalities between writer and readers through reference to scarred bodies marking communal membership.

Disciplined and mirrored body types. Although stories of restitution include healthcare providers as narrative features, they put the responsibility of behavior change and "staying clean" on themselves. Phrases such as "I forced myself to stop" and "I've let myself feel my emotions" establish agency and control over the situation so that staying clean is ultimately a matter of will power. Such stories are about disciplining oneself, despite otherwise uncontrollable events swirling around them—a breakup, loss of a job, and so forth. Restitution narratives in the sample are hopeful assertions illustrating that safer coping mechanisms can be found, probably necessitating medical help, but that the strength to do so must come from oneself.

Offering themselves as role models, writers of restitution narratives affirm that choosing a safer alternative to self-injury is a matter of personal choice and responsibility. While never cajoling or condemning readers, restitution narratives make clear through gentle encouragement that Redditors who currently self-injure *can* decide to seek help and *can* choose to find alternative means of handling the chaos swirling around them if they want to.

QUEST NARRATIVE

Only one story qualifies as a quest narrative in the sample. The entry is, by far, the longest in the sample. The first half is the backstory describing how the writer began self-injuring and ultimately managed to stop. The second half consists of five detailed "lessons I've learnt along this journey." Titled "Addiction Sucks," the story features three basic chapters that Frank compares with "the hero's quest" as described by mythologist, Joseph Campbell (1949). In the first chapter, what Frank calls the "departure" (1995/2013, p. 117), the writer explains:

> I cut for the first time when I was 14 and my mum found out very quickly which made me stop for a while. I had some more flare ups when I was 16.

Mention of the author's mother is significant, illustrating a breach between maternal normalcy and aberrant adolescent cutting.

The second chapter—the "initiation" (Frank 1995/2013, p. 118)—is very brief, referring to a period of addiction and a shift in self-identification from son to addict: "What I didn't realize and what nobody told me is that self harm is incredibly addictive and that an addiction stays with you."

The final chapter is "return" marked by transformative "apotheosis:" "The teller returns as one who is no longer ill but remains marked by illness [and] has been given something by the experience, usually some insight that must be passed on to others" (Frank 1995/2013, p. 118). This is the longest part of the narrative in which the author refers to hearing a song about climbing up from a low point:

> I eventually managed to stop myself from cutting with a promise . . . I told myself that I would never be as low as I had been if I could make sure I was safe in my own head and wouldn't hurt myself. It hasn't always worked but I have had something to hold onto in my darkest times.

Desire, contingency, and control are neatly condensed into this short passage. Desire is for an end of cutting; however, the lure of cutting is always present. Control is focused on the self and the disciplined body.

As shown among restitution narratives, this writer has taken particular care not to force their views on readers. This is not a story about domination, but about communicating alternatives, offering oneself as a model—again, an exemplar of the mirroring body:

> If you're struggling or dont know how to start getting better then I dont want this to discourage or depress you. I am telling you what I wish I was told. Too many people will tell you "it gets better" or other platitudes. The shitty truth is that only you can dig yourself out of this hole. Outside help is fantastic and can facilitate a recovery but it comes from you.

The responsibility for change is once more ultimately left to the reader as with restitution narratives.

Association with the body is difficult to ascertain in this story. References to cutting and to himself suggest that the author drifts from end to end of the association/dissociation continuum. The author refers to *cutting* himself five times, and yet, never mentions where he cut on his body; this suggests that the particular place on the body is unimportant because cutting anywhere is cutting oneself. On the other hand, when describing *other forms* of self-injury, the writer does distinguish between the acting self and the body part as if they were independent:

> I have beaten my head against desks and punched my fist through a wall. However I dont fully count these incidents, I dont know why but it's different when it's a cut. Its sharper and it tastes like ice. But I can forgive myself for these slip ups.

For this person, cutting is qualitatively different from other forms of self-injury with regard to perception and experience.

While "Addiction Sucks" has all the markings of a quest narrative, it is also indicative of why narrative analysis is always tentative and interpretive. Like most stories told "in the field," this one doesn't totally conform to academic models because of the author's distinction between cutting and other manifestations of self-harm—a distinction that clinicians might find difficult to accept. From this writer's perspective, cutting is in a category of its own; other forms of self-injury are dangerous, just not to the extent of cutting. Adopting the writer's perspective, we can say that the quest to overcome *cutting* was successful, although other forms of self-injury persist.

Also, contrary to the tidier quest narrative exemplars presented by Frank, for this storyteller, the journey is not yet complete. Contingency is still a reality, as revealed in the closing lines:

> I hope this isn't too bleak. I do genuinely feel optimistic about the future about 50% of the time. I just want to let you all know. I'm still here 9 years on and 7 years clean. It's hard but I'm surviving.

As this example demonstrates, stories are not neat packages. In fact, they are rather leaky vessels, with elements oozing from one category to another. The writer, in this case, looks backward with some degree of satisfaction, but remains less sanguine about the future. He walks a fine line between being clean and resuming cutting, while other forms of self-injury are always a possibility.

ABSENT BODY TYPE

So far, we have examined all three forms of illness narratives in Frank's model. Within the stories presented here, we have also seen three of the four body types described in Frank's typology: disciplined bodies, communicative bodies, and mirroring bodies.

The absence of the fourth body type in Frank's model—the dominating body—is worthy of consideration. Given that people sometimes turn to self-injury as a form of self-punishment, it is possible that those who self-injure are simply not the type of people who would try to dominate others in the ways that Frank describes. They might prefer to seek domination via discipline and punishment with respect to their own bodies rather than to control the bodies of others.

Indeed, as we have already seen, writers specifically emphasize that they are *not* trying to control other people, whether that be family members, friends, or other Redditors. One person, for example, explains that having stopped self-harming, they are feeling emotions that they haven't felt for months. Unfortunately, that leads to new problems in relating to their parents:

> They always pretend everything is okay, and that like im okay, but im not and i dont think they understand how hard it is to stay clean everyday with all this shit that im starting to feel again. i just with they knew, but i dont know how to tell them without like either them getting mad at me for being upset or i start getting upset because im a literal fucking crybaby now and lose what im trying to say.

This writer is reluctant to challenge parental denial and, thus, to force their parents to face the problem.

The closest instance to a dominating body is found in one story where the writer tries to avoid control by others via deception:

> school nurse found out i cut so it got to my parents, now they watch me all the time I'm lying to her making her think im fine now until she lets me stop going
> then ill start again , and im okay with it

This is one of only two posts in the sample in which the writers seem comfortable with self-injury, exhibiting no evident feelings of remorse or desire to change. Deception is, arguably, a means toward control through construction of a false story; however, the manipulation is not to get anyone to do anything. Rather, in this situation, deception is used to regain agency for oneself—to regain control over the ability to seek pleasure and relief from internal stress via self-injury.

DISCUSSION

Stories in r/selfharm provide a rich source of data pertaining to perspectives, opinions, attitudes, beliefs, and behaviors among an online community of people who self-injure. Although we cannot infer much about demographics because of Reddit's constraints necessarily protecting anonymity, the same conditions permit safety among writers to tell stories in their own voices without fear of retribution. As such, stories shared in r/selfharm are vivid, detailed, and deeply thoughtful in their descriptions of social context, emotions, memories, desires, ambitions, and even physical sensations associated with self-injury, in particular, and their lives more generally. And because there are so many stories produced on a daily basis, this chapter has only provided a glimpse into the abundance of data available—a small snapshot of the ongoing narrative flow.

Dominant narratives and contextual biases. As we have seen, following Frank's illness narrative model, most narratives collected in the sample can be classified as chaos narratives. This dominant mode of storytelling illustrates in form and content the overwhelming internal and external conflicts conditioning self-injury. Stories of recovery—that is, restitution and quest narratives—are far fewer in number. The imbalance between chaos narratives and restitution/quest narratives reveal that the paramount concern in r/selfharm is to express what is happening in the present, sometimes even in the moment. Less frequent restitution/quest narratives take a longer view through time, looking backward to where the writers came from and, only occasionally, forward toward a better future.

Emphasis on present crises is, again, a function of the channel of communication. Social media such as Reddit, to borrow Innis' (1951) term is "biased" toward the momentary and the ephemeral. Despite the fact that posts are archived, they are written in the moment, often lasting at the top of the discussion for just a few minutes before gradually moving downward into the past.

This temporal bias helps explain the notable difference in findings between what is reported in this chapter and earlier research described by Amy Chandler (2014), also using Frank's typology. In fact, Chandler found the exact opposite among her interviews with people who self-injured in the past. For Chandler, quest stories were the most commonly told narratives, and chaos stories were the least abundant. Chandler suggested that her finding could have been due to the context of the storytelling as her participants were asked about self-injury within larger "life-story" discussions. It is possible, Chandler (p. 115) points out that "the nature and setting of the research interview encourages particular forms of narrative . . . and there may have been an impulse in providing such an account to give a positive ending." In narrative analysis, context and channel condition narrative content, so it should not be surprising to find that stories told in one context vary widely from those in another context.

Body types and problems of embodiment. Frank's model is more than a typology of three narrative types, as each story reveals nuanced perspectives on how storytellers see, feel, and relate to their bodies. As demonstrated above, harm inflicted upon the body is variously framed in terms of necessity, rebellion, shame, pride, and remorse. The body is used sometimes as a medium through which cutting, burning, and other self-injurious methods are means of comforting oneself in times of confusion and internal struggle. Less often, bodies marked in the past are used to make a case for overcoming the desire to self-injure now, with a hopeful—but never guaranteed—message of a brighter future.

Contrary to what Frank predicts in *The Wounded Storyteller*, a consistent pattern runs through all three forms of narrative in this chapter pertaining to the theme of desire. If desire is demand for more of something, that something in these stories is *control*. Whether writers describe chaos, restitution, or quest, their repeated refrain is a longing—if not a demand—for control over conditions in which they live, including familial support and respect, dependable friendships, and unfavorable judgments by healthcare providers, teachers, counselors, and other authority figures.

Storytellers posting in r/selfharm also want control over themselves. With the exception of two writers who seemed quite comfortable with cutting, that means being able to find other means of handling conflict and anxiety that are *less efficacious* than self-injury. I stress this point because this is the conundrum faced by people who self-injure: For many, self-injury *works* as Levitt notes in chapter 2 of this book. It does the job of easing frustration, anger, and fear, but I must emphasize, *in the moment*.

Again, discourse in r/selfharm is primarily about the past or the present. For the person who actively self-injures, the future seems a long way off. Yet if self-injury is affective in the moment, it is also a source of self-blame and ultimately, implication of weakness. Writers in r/selfharm repeatedly curse themselves for cutting, burning, and so forth, yet they also know that, to some extent, self-injury is effective. They thus live what in Burke (1961) famously termed the "guilt-redemption cycle," lamenting their perceived weakness amid a culture that values individualism and self-discipline, yet unable to otherwise cope with external, unpredictable forces.

Among the narratives examined here, self-injury is not atonement for imperfection as one might assume. Rather it's *evidence of* imperfection, adding to the burden of anxiety already created by familial conflict and other external factors, now weighted even more by stigma. Paradoxically, self-injury is also an effective mode of escape. Hence, the cycle of self-injury and self-blame goes around and around.

A few Redditors find their way out of the cycle, but stay in the discursive community of r/selfharm (or return after an absence) to encourage others to find their own means of escape. Escape from the cycle, however, is always conditional, as participants who have not self-injured for months, or even years, describe an ongoing desire to resume self-harming.

Community. Early in this chapter, I defined r/selfharm as a platform. Given the evidence presented here, it is more than that. Like so many forums, r/selfharm is a channel through which imagined community is constructed through discourse. It serves as a "public sphere" (Habermas 1961/1991) created by and for people who self-harm who would not have the opportunity to gather face-to-face. If Frank's model tells us anything, it's that the self-injury community is far from monolithic.

By far, most communal members currently self-injure, living lives of quiet desperation amid circumstances that, for them, are defined by chaos and lack of agency. A second, much smaller, group expresses itself through restitution and quest narratives. Rather than focus primarily on a tumultuous present, they tend to look backward, measuring past self-injury against tentative alternative means of handling chaos in the present. Their goal is to encourage others and to offer themselves as models of survival. They are careful not to demand or promise too much, for they, like their more numerous communal counterparts, recognize uncontrollable contingency that conditions their lives.

CONCLUSION

Self-injury is never normalized in stories we have examined here. Rather, it is secretive and contrary to dominant, socially sanctioned behavior. As such, even though self-injury serves a valuable purpose as a coping mechanism, it is recognized as a social taboo even by those who engage in it. Further, storytellers realize that, despite its positive effects, self-injury is physically dangerous.

Because self-injury is simultaneously taboo, hazardous, *and* seen as an effective means of handling stress, there is no easy way to end the cycle. Why would one surrender a means of handling trouble that seems to work so well? On the other hand, why continue a practice that is socially condemned and life threatening?

In this chapter, I have tried to listen deeply to self-injury stories by using tools offered via narrative analysis. I have looked for emergent patterns across stories to reveal shared ways that writers experience their lives and the world around them, and I have examined common themes relating to storytellers' beliefs and attitudes about self-injury in its many forms. This chapter, however, is not without limitations.

First, my sample is small. I began with hundreds of stories comprising the entire population of stories told in one week. Such a large sample was overwhelming for qualitative analysis, and I decided that a smaller sample would allow me to dig deeper into the stories. The cost, however, is obvious in that fifty stories cannot be said to adequately describe the thousands of stories told yearly on r/selfharm. Future researchers could use Frank's model on a much larger number of stories, perhaps looking for meaningful statistical relationships among narrative categories and other variables such as modes of self-injury, semantic patterns, and so forth.

Second, as a lone researcher, I was quite comfortable using an interpretive approach; however, others might question why I coded stories into one category as opposed to another. The interpretive scholar's answer to such questions is to simply say that I have made my case, supporting my observations and conclusions with empirical data. Other scholars might want to test my conclusions further by taking a more quantitative approach, for example, using multiple coders to test for reliability.

The biggest limitation in this study is that I did not examine responses to stories told. Communication is transactional and interactive rather than a one-way, linear process. The give and take between storytellers and their audience is crucial in fully understanding how discourse about self-injury functions. I hope that this chapter piques the interest of other researchers who will pick up where I left off by examining how readers respond to stories, and further yet, how storytellers engage with their respondents.

WORKS CITED

American Psychiatric Association. *Diagnostic and Statistical Manual of Mental Disorders* (5th ed.). Arlington, VA: American Psychiatric Publishing, 2013.

Anderson, Benedict. *Imagined Communities: Reflections on the Origin and Spread of Nationalism.* London: Verso Books, 1983.

Bar-On, Vered. "It Cuts Both Ways: An Analysis of the Psychological Discourse on Self-Injury from a Linguistic Point of View." *The Psychoanalytic Review* 101, no. 5 (2014): 701–734.

Burke, Kenneth. *The Rhetoric of Religion: Studies in Logology.* Berkeley: University of California Press, 1961.

Campbell, Joseph. *The Hero with a Thousand Faces.* Princeton: Bollingen Foundation, 1949.

Chandler, Amy. "Inviting Pain? Pain, Dualism and Embodiment in Narratives of Self-Injury." *Sociology of Health & Illness* 35 (2013): 716–730.

Chandler, Amy. "Narrating the Self-Injured Body." *Medical Humanities* 40 (2014): 111–116.

Charon, Rita. *Narrative Medicine: Honoring the Stories of Illness.* New York: Oxford University Press, 2006.

Charon, Rita, and Martha Montello (Eds.). *Stories Matter: The Role of Narrative in Medical Ethics.* New York: Routledge, 2002.

Eliseo-Arras, Rebecca K., Rachel Brous, and Sandra M. Sheppard. "A Content and Thematic Analysis of Tumblr Posts Related to Non-Suicidal Self-Injury." *Journal of Ethnographic & Qualitative Research* 13 (2019): 198–211.

Frank, Arthur W. "From Dysappearance to Hyperappearance: Sliding Boundaries of Illness and Bodies." In *The Body and Psychology*, edited by Henderikus J. Stam. Thousand Oaks, CA: Sage, 1998.

Frank, Arthur W. *The Wounded Storyteller: Body, Illness, and Ethics.* Chicago: University of Chicago Press, 2013. (Original work published in 1995).
Geertz, Clifford. *The Interpretation of Cultures.* New York: Basic Books, 1973.
Habermas, Jurgen. *The Structural Transformation of the Public Sphere: An Inquiry into a Category of Bourgeois Society,* translated by Thomas Burger with Frederick Lawrence. Cambridge, MA: MIT Press, 1991. (Original work published in 1961).
Horner, Gail. "Nonsuicidal Self-Injury." *Journal of Pediatric Health Care* 30 (2016): 261–267.
Hoyos, Carlos, Vencent Mancini, Yulia Furlong, Nick Medford, Hugo Critchley, and Wai Chen. "The Role of Dissociation and Abuse Among Adolescents Who Self-Harm." *Australian & New Zealand Journal of Psychiatry* 53 (2019): 989–999.
Hyvarinen, Matti. "Analyzing Narrative Genres." In *The Handbook of Narrative Analysis,* edited by Anna De Fina and Alexandra Georgakopoulou, 178–193. Hoboken, NJ: Wiley, 2015.
In-Albon, Tina, Claudia Ruf, and Marc Schmid. "Proposed Diagnostic Criteria for the *DSM-5* of Nonsuicidal Self-Injury in Female Adolescents: Diagnostic and Clinical Correlates." *Psychiatry Journal* (2013): Article ID 159208.
Innis, Harold. *The Bias of Communication.* Toronto: University of Toronto Press, 1951.
Kelly, Michael P., and Hilary Dickinson. "The Narrative Self in Autobiographical Accounts of Illness." *The Sociological Review* 45 (1997): 254–278.
Kleinman, Arthur. *The Illness Narratives: Suffering, Healing, and the Human Condition.* New York: Basic Books, 1988.
Labov, William, and Joshua Waletzky. "Narrative Analysis: Oral Versions of Personal Experience." In *Essays on Verbal and Visual Arts,* edited by June Helm, 12–44. Seattle: University of Washington Press.
Marshall, Harriette, and Anjum Yazdani. "Locating Culture in Accounting for Self-Harm Amongst Asian Young Women." *Journal of Community & Applied Social Psychology* 9 (1999): 413–433.
Memon, Aksha M., Shiva G. Sharma, Satyajit S. Mohite, and Shailesh Jain. "The Role of Online Social Networking on Deliberate Self-Harm and Suicidality in Adolescents: A Systematized Review of Literature." *Indian Journal of Psychiatry* 60 (2018): 384–392.
Murray, Michael. "A Narrative Approach to Health Psychology: Background and Potential." *Journal of Health Psychology* 2 (1997): 9–20.
Paris, Joel. "Understanding Self-Mutilation in Borderline Personality Disorder." *Harvard Review of Psychiatry* 13 (2005): 179–185.
Riessman, Catherine. "Performing Identities in Illness Narrative: Masculinity and Multiple Sclerosis." *Qualitative Research* 3 (2003): 5–33.
Riessman, Catherine Kohler. *Narrative Analysis.* Newbury Park: Sage Publications, 1993.
Seko, Yukari, Sean A. Kidd, David Wiljer, and Kwame J. McKenzie. "On the Creative Edge: Exploring Motivations for Creating Non-Suicidal Self-Injury Content Online." *Qualitative Health Research* 25 (2015): 1334–1346.

Seko, Yukari, and Stephen P. Lewis. "The Self-Harmed, Visualized, and Reblogged: Remaking of Self-Injury Narratives on Tumblr." *New Media & Society* 20 (2018): 180–198.

Seymour-Smith, Sarah, and Margaret Weatherell. "'What He Hasn't Told You...': Investigating the Micro-Politics of Gendered Support in Heterosexual Couples' Co-Constructed Accounts of Illness." *Feminism and Psychology* 16 (2006): 105–127.

Shimazono, Yosuke. *Narrative Analysis in Medical Anthropology.* Diss., Institute of Social and Cultural Anthropology, University of Oxford, 2003.

Sinclair, Julia, and Judith Green, J. "Understanding Resolution of Deliberate Self Harm: Qualitative Interview Study of Patients' Experiences." *BMJ: British Medical Journal* 330, no. 7500 (2005): 1112–1115.

Wiseman, Justin Michael. *Self-Compassion and Its Relation to Nonsuicidal Self-Injury.* Diss., The Wright School of Professional Psychology, Wright State University, 2018.

Zetterqvist, Maria. "The DSM-5 Diagnosis of Nonsuicidal Self-Injury Disorder: A Review of the Empirical Literature." *Child and Adolescent Psychiatry and Mental Health* 9 (2015): 31.

Chapter 8

Fighting the Self

Interpersonal and Intrapersonal Communicative Violence in Chuck Palahniuk's Fight Club

Lisann Anders

"The barrel of the gun pressed against the back of my throat, Tyler says, 'We really won't die'" (Palahniuk 1996, 11). The second paragraph of Chuck Palahniuk's *Fight Club* already states what the novel is about. It is about violence, but it is also about survival through violence. This tension provides one of the core paradigms that is constantly communicated and negotiated within the text. Violence in *Fight Club* is predominantly physical. It revolves around the body as the center of violence, as both the violator and the violated, thus being transformed into a tool that is supposed to free the mind.

This freedom of mind can be seen in the Narrator's creation of his imagined alter-ego Tyler Durden. Tyler is the one who blows up the Narrator's apartment and founds Fight Club in order to make the Narrator feel alive through physical pain and suffering. It is what Freud coined the "oceanic feeling," a "oneness with the universe" that "seeks to reinstate limitless narcissism" (Freud 2010, 21). It is this wholeness of the self which is sought for and which lays the basis for Fight Club. The latter creates a community for the Narrator, a setting, in which he can feel complete and in control through the individual fights. Therefore, the various Fight Clubs represent a platform of communication for men. Here, they can express themselves and be free by means of injuring each other.

It can thus be argued that the body in pain becomes the essence of communication. However, this communication is not just experienced on an interpersonal level because the violence also takes place internally, that is, within the Narrator, who fights against Tyler. Hence, through Tyler and the Fight Clubs, the Narrator learns to communicate. Since Tyler and the Narrator share a body, the violence can be seen as intrapersonal, it is directed against the self, which highlights the Narrator's inner struggle. Therefore, this chapter will argue that the text presents a form of non-suicidal self-injury (NSSI), which is used as a form of intrapersonal communication to establish interpersonal communication and relationships. I would like to explore how violence and injuries play a liberating role in the novel, *Fight Club*, by helping men communicate with each other. At the same time, the communicative function of self-injurious behaviors also leads to risks and consequences. Furthermore, I would like to explore why it is only men who can communicate through injuries in the text and what the role of the female is in this masculine world. Chuck Palahniuk's novel will be the main focus of my discussion; however, David Fincher's 1999 film adaptation, starring Edward Norton and Brad Pitt, also influences considerations and representations taken into account in this discussion of self-injury as communication.

NSSI: NON-SUICIDAL SELF-INJURY

Before going into detail about self-injury as a communicative process, the concept of NSSI needs to be considered more thoroughly. NSSI aims at harming one's own body without committing suicide. It is the physical pain that is foregrounded. The most common form of NSSI is probably cutting; however, burning and beating oneself provide other means to injure the body. Matthew Nock (2009) defines NSSI as the "direct, deliberate destruction of one's own body tissue in the absence of intent to die" (78). The emphasis on the deliberate intention of pain is crucial here as it is different from physical effects of drug consumption. The reason for the self-injury can often be found in a discontent with the self (on an intrapersonal level) or a disharmonious external situation caused by interpersonal conflicts (Nock 2009, 79). Self-injury is a means to deal with "emotional stress, [for] self-punishment, [to] escape from unpleasant circumstances, [for] gaining attention, and escape from a feeling of bodily and emotional numbness" (Bareiss 2017, 319). NSSI is thus used as escapism in order to flee from an unpleasant reality and instances "of self-injury are shown to be closely tied to socio-cultural contexts" (Chandler 2012, 443). Interestingly enough, even though NSSI is not bound to gender and can be found in all age groups, the practice of self-harm is, in its cultural discourse, assumed to be gendered and believed to be spread more among women, usually adolescent females (Gilman 2013, 150). According to Chris Millard, it "is an activity principally by those gendered female, and that the stereotyped behavior involves cutting the skin" (2013, 128). It is this self-mutilation that provides these female "self-cutters" with an identity (ibid., 137). Millard refers to Adler and Adler's study, *The Tender Cut* (2011), when describing the distinction between people who "invent" self-injury for themselves as a means of creating an identity—generally, prior to 1996—and those who find their identity as someone who self-injures in the imitation by others after 1996 who learned the behavior via media or friends (Millard 2013, 137). This shift might have been influenced by the change in communication through the new medium of the Internet and the introduction of the messaging service ICQ in 1996 and the overall increase of Internet access in that year (Shedden 1996).

This distinction of invention and imitation of NSSI can also be observed in Chuck Palahniuk's novel *Fight Club*. Published in 1996—the pivotal year noted by Millard and Shedden, respectively—it parallels the shift in those who self-injure that invent themselves and those who follow. The novel, as well as the movie by David Fincher, depicts the invention of a club for the purpose of the physical destruction of the male body. Gender stereotypes of self-harm are thus reversed by the founder of this Fight Club, Tyler Durden, the hallucinated double of the Narrator, who attempts to rebel against society's emasculating capitalism. This emasculation is also reminiscent of the emasculated male body in the novel represented by the testicular cancer support group "Remaining Men Together." The support group of Tyler Durden's Fight Club is thus also concerned with the preservation of masculinity. Here, in order to be men, communication is taken from the level of the verbal component to the level of body language. Albeit verbal communication about the club is forbidden, rumors spread and consequently, men, join the club because they have heard of it and are intrigued by the idea of harming themselves and each other to gain a sense of control again over their bodies and their masculinity.

Nock (2009) identifies several processes that trigger NSSI:

> A functional approach suggests that NSSI is maintained by several reinforcement processes: intrapersonal negative reinforcement (i.e., NSSI decreases or distracts from aversive thoughts or feelings), intrapersonal positive reinforcement (i.e., NSSI generates desired feelings or stimulation), interpersonal positive reinforcement (i.e., NSSI facilitates help-seeking), or interpersonal negative reinforcement (i.e., NSSI facilitates escape from undesired social situations). (79)

These processes can indeed be applied to Palahniuk's novel (and Fincher's film, respectively) and they will serve as a structuring element in the following for the discussion of NSSI and *Fight Club*.

INTRAPERSONAL NEGATIVE REINFORCEMENT

Faking Injuries to Communicate

Even though the novel begins with a gun in the Narrator's mouth, hinting at a potential suicide—or rather, murder (at that point we do not know about the Narrator's split personality), the first form of self-injury we encounter in the story can be found in the support groups the Narrator is attending. Drawing on the film, Tracey Parker (2008) explains that movies such as *Fight Club* "interrogate but do not undermine self-help culture and its commodification in their subject matter, and each film reinforces the fragmentation of the individual through fragmented narratives and style" (2). This fragmentation of narrative is also apparent in the structure of the novel, but even further emphasized in its content. Here, a fragmentation of reality can be observed from the very beginning. The Narrator suffers from insomnia, which often includes a distortion of reality or as the Narrator describes it himself, "an out-of-body experience" (Palahniuk 1996, 19); yet, the major fragmentation can be seen in the Narrator's personality as he becomes schizophrenic. Before he loses his sense of reality, though, the Narrator tries to cure his insomnia and consults a doctor to get some sedatives; however, the latter does not treat the Narrator's condition seriously and advises him to stop by some cancer support groups to see "real" pain.

This is interesting in so far as the Narrator suffers from the lack of sleep, but there are no physical signs for his pain, which is why the communication between the Narrator and his doctor fails. This already hints at a need for an outer appearance of pain in order to be turned into interpersonal communication as well as interpersonal positive reinforcement, that is, the seeking for help through visible wounds, be it in the form of bruises and cuts or other forms of bodily changes.

Interpersonal communication is thus not possible at this stage since the pain is intrapersonal, that is, psychological. The sleeping problems are not a form of NSSI yet, but the failure of interpersonal communication between doctor and patient leads the Narrator to NSSI in the form of faked pain in the support groups. By pretending to be sick, the Narrator fake-injures himself, that is, he pretends to have a disease even though he is physically healthy, and thus distracts himself from his internal problems that have caused his insomnia, which is why the support groups can be regarded as a form of intrapersonal negative reinforcement. This should not diminish the validity of group therapy, but the Narrator cannot truly relate to the suffering of the support group members. According to Nock (2009),

> People may escalate to the use of NSSI as a means of communication when less intense strategies (e.g., speaking, yelling) have failed due to poor signal or

clarity, or when such strategies have not produced the desired effect due to an unresponsive or invalidating environment. (80)

Spoken language does thus not suffice to achieve communication and understanding; it has to be substituted by a more physical communication—a kind of nonverbal communication. Thus, it is ironic that the doctor, who is supposed to ease pain, encourages the Narrator, to some degree at least, to experience "real pain" (19). The support groups revolve around people who are gradually dying and suffer bodily pain such as brain parasites or testicular cancer. These two groups are interesting in themselves as the brain parasites group foreshadows Tyler Durden, who can be regarded as a parasite eating up the Narrator; whereas testicular cancer with its telling group name, "Remaining Men Together," hints at the loss of masculinity the Narrator is experiencing and which later has to be compensated by the overly masculine Tyler.

Distraction from Social Emasculation

The loss of masculinity manifests itself already in the Narrator's sleeping problems, as he lacks control over his body, but it can also be observed on a social level where the "body has been sliced out of modern life and reduced to a consuming good" (Burgess 2012, 270). James Craine and Stuart Aitken (2004) argue that

> insomnia, [is] a symptom often associated with societal pressures, and he [the Narrator] creates an alter-ego to cope [. . .]. Jack [the Narrator] reacts to, and is mobilized by, his inability to exist in a masculinity society delineated by consumption—he becomes alienated entering the homosocial and homoerotic world of Tyler, his monstrous doppelgaenger. (292)

The Narrator defines himself by consumer goods such as **IKEA** furniture and his job as a recall specialist, in which he has to evaluate consumer goods. He tries to control his lifestyle by following interior design trends, and he tries to control consumer goods in his job—thus distracting himself from the feeling of emasculation without being aware of reinforcing it by means of his opportunistic behavior. He fails, however, on both levels.

This failure of what is perceived as being masculine in a postmodern capitalist society is rooted in the Narrator's lack of interpersonal communication as well as physical contact. That is the reason why the Narrator finds comfort in the support groups, "where the instability and suffering he witnesses dispel his own alienation. His insomnia is a kind of disease, separating him from immediately experienced life" (Burgess 2006, 270). The groups are not only about trauma reprocessing, the sharing of suffering, or death, but also about physical contact, such as hugging. They provide a space which serves as an emotional outlet for the group members. Their physical pain is thus supposed to be eased by breaking down emotional boundaries and expressing one's feelings.

Since the Narrator is not experiencing physical pain, for him, the support groups can be seen as a form of self-injury on an imaginary level. His pretending of diseases is a form of self-harm that only happens in his mind and not on a physical level. It is only "[e]xhausted bodies and hysterical language [that] *are* the opportunities for change, and it is with the body that discourse becomes even possible" (ibid., 267, original emphasis). The Narrator's body, however, is not exhausted; it is not decaying, and yet, he pretends that it is. This pretense of physical suffering can be seen as an inner longing for pain in order to feel more alive as the diseases are at least "reminders of the body's *existence*" (ibid., 271, original emphasis). By creating a proximity to death, the Narrator tries to experience what it is like to live, which includes interpersonal relationships, physical contact, and emotions: "This is better than real life. [. . .] Every evening I died, and every evening I was born. Resurrected. *Until tonight*" (Palahniuk 1996, 22, emphasis added).

INTERPERSONAL POSITIVE REINFORCEMENT

Marla Singer as the Trigger for NSSI

The Narrator's self-inflicted, would-be diseases do not work anymore once Marla Singer shows up and identifies him as a fraud

> Marla Singer [. . .] disrupts the cycle of death and resurrection. Marla's presence reminds him that he is himself seeking authenticity by copying others; he is not sick but he can copy being sick. (Burgess 2012, 271)

Like the Narrator, Marla Singer attends the multiple support groups without being sick. She is a woman who suddenly appears and poses a threat to the Narrator's pretense game. She can be seen as another double to the Narrator as her behavior often mirrors his. Furthermore, she enters a romantic, or at least physical, relationship with Tyler Durden—and by extension with the Narrator. Once Marla appears, the Narrator's pretense of bodily suffering deflates, and the mental suffering in the form of sleeplessness returns. This time, the Narrator cannot escape into the safety of imagined injuries. Instead, he compensates the loss of the support groups by a support group of his own.

In that way, Marla can be regarded as an interpersonal positive reinforcement since her appearance leads the Narrator to imagine Tyler Durden, which can be seen as a subconscious act of self-harm (after all, schizophrenia is not really a healthy coping mechanism due to its rather incontrollable nature), which leads him to found the support group that he coins "Fight Club." Tyler is the Narrator's new support, his new guidance, and in a way, his new doctor. The prescription—or rather, self-medication, is to found a support group for men only in order to experience real pain as well as masculine bonding, a space which "allows the Narrator to transition from mimicking pain and otherness to embodying it" (Burgess 2012, 271). The support group Fight Club, which can be seen as a brand of its own, is created; it is a group in which females are excluded (cf. Craine and Aitken 2004, 293), thus automatically linking masculinity to violence and pain.

INTERPERSONAL NEGATIVE REINFORCEMENT

Reclaiming Masculinity through NSSI

Ironically, as outlined before, NSSI is often associated with females in medical scholarship, but *Fight Club* shows males who self-injure trying to reclaim their masculinity through this culturally connoted female behavior which already foreshadows the failure of violent masculinity. Burgess (2012) argues that to "escape a life that is outwardly 'complete' but inwardly numbing, the Narrator in the novel invents the community of Fight Club, where brutal fist fights, injuries, and pain instantly jolt the participants back into an immediate connection with primal, fully embodied, and, according to their principles, more genuine existence" (265).

Fight Club represents a support group that does not deal with "accidental" pain in the form of diseases, but it focuses on self-inflicted pain as a form of escape mechanism from the individual everyday problems of the club's members. This physical pain has, however, also a socio-psychological dimension to it. The members of Fight Club suffer from a loss of masculinity resulting in isolation and alienation within a consumerist society in which goods matter more than people, in which everything is unified and an individual identity is impossible. Craine and Aitken (2004) describe this loss as "the crisis of masculinity [which] is in large part about the marginalization of men" (289). Hence, what men in general and the Narrator, in particular, try to achieve in the novel is to gain access to the center again, to create a male identity. To them, "[m]ale violence offers men a performative basis on which to construct masculine identity" (Giroux 2001, 19).

In this case, this male violence is expressed through a form of self-injury, generating identification with the violence itself (Nock 2009, 81). The men in *Fight Club* want a life within which they are the protagonist, where they are the leading figure, and where they are in control. In the quasi-support group Fight Club, the Narrator as well as each participant sees "a cure of what ails him personally, a meaningless life of consumerism and conformism" (Irwin 2013, 677). This cure through NSSI is communicated interpersonally through physical interaction between the group members. It is also negatively reinforced, primarily serving as an escape mechanism from the individual as well as general social situation—feeling physical pain instead of psychological or social pain.

INTRAPERSONAL POSITIVE REINFORCEMENT

Feeling Oneself through NSSI

Like NSSI more generally, Fight Club is practiced in secrecy (Chandler 2012, 443). Of course, it is ironic that the men's motivation for being themselves is undermined by the fact that Fight Club "remains underground and the men begin to lead double lives" (Parker 2008, 8). Instead of constructing one whole life, members of Fight Club choose a split life. The Narrator "chooses" a split personality that reflects the double-sidedness of NSSI—the hidden performance of self harm and the pretense of normality in public.

Fight Club can thus be seen as not only a place for NSSI, but also a metaphor for self-harm. It is a secret practice, and it harms its members physically. It is also a means of generating desired feelings of freedom and masculinity, thus presenting it as intrapersonal or, rather, intra-social positive reinforcement of the masculinity crisis.

Likewise, Tyler Durden grants the Narrator a sense of masculine power, using NSSI in a more literal way. The Narrator beats himself up even though it seems as if he is fighting with Tyler, but since they share a body, it can be considered as a way of self-harm. This fight scene between Tyler and the Narrator, in particular, presents a form of intrapersonal positive reinforcement. This stimulation is even more foregrounded when Tyler imprints a chemical burn on the Narrator's hand (Palahniuk 1996, 73–78) as a form of "guided meditation they use at support groups" (ibid., 75). Because burning is a form of NSSI that is frequently used by individuals who self-injure, meditation and self-injury as a means of communicating with the self are equated.

Feeling One through NSSI

The same chemical burns that the Narrator receives, or is rather inflicting on himself, are also given to the members of Fight Club, what the Narrator calls

"Tyler's kiss" (ibid., 177). They are given a sense of belonging by chosen pain, a pain that is to give them a new sense of life and a new sense of community. Therefore, in order to feel themselves as individuals as well as a group—in order to feel alive—they need a physical outlet to remember that they are still there, that they are still men. Burgess (2012, 267) emphasizes that a "community structured around the body is not necessarily an escape from thought and reason but another and perhaps more productive path toward awareness." This awareness of the self is what Fight Club aims at with its physicality and brutality, providing its members a stimulating feeling of masculinity and power over the self. In this way, the definition of self-injury can be broadened because the men do not cut or hit themselves, but, rather, position themselves in the club to be beaten up.

REINFORCEMENT PROCESSES COMBINED

Communicating Social Problems through Violence

The participants come to the club because it is their way of stating that something is wrong in their lives outside the group. Using violence against the self as a form of communicating psychological problems of the self is even taken a step further and set in a social context by means of Project Mayhem wherein the individual body is augmented to the social body. Project Mayhem is an extension of Fight Club. It is a quasi-religious organization with the purpose of openly opposing and attacking societal norms by means of extreme violence against people who conform to the social system. "While Fight Club uses consensual violence to gain an immediate sense of liberation, Project Mayhem directs violence outwards to nonconsenting others and justifies its actions by the promise of liberation in the future" (Burgess 2012, 268). Project Mayhem can, therefore, be regarded as the fascist mission Tyler sets up to hurt the capitalist system, analogously represented in the destruction of the male body.

Intrapersonal Processes of NSSI in Project Mayhem

Committing a form of social self-harm as buildings are destroyed and society is targeted, Project Mayhem can be regarded as an extended means of NSSI. Indeed, individuals who are not part of the project are threatened with violence and are mentally tortured by being held at gun-point like Raymond Hessel (Palahniuk 1996, 151–155) or held captive and menaced with castration as in the case of the police commissioner (ibid., 164–166). Because these individuals comprise part of the social body, that is, society outside Fight Club, the claim for NSSI can be made on a metaphorical level. Therefore, this kind of NSSI can be seen as intrapersonal and positively reinforced as it tries to achieve a desired feeling, namely freedom from social norms through self-injury. With Project Mayhem, Tyler Durden aims at fighting what Slavoj Žižek (2009) calls "systemic violence" by "subjective violence" (2). Žižek describes the systemic, societal violence by explaining that "We're talking here of the violence inherent in a system: not only direct physical violence, but also the more subtle forms of coercion that sustain relations of domination and exploitation, including the threat of violence" (8). It is this domination Tyler has in mind when initiating Project Mayhem:

> When Tyler invented Project Mayhem, Tyler said the goal of Project Mayhem had nothing to do with other people. Tyler didn't care if other people got hurt or not. The goal was to teach each man in the project that he had the power to control history. We, each of us, can take control of the world. (Palahniuk 1996, 122)

While an attempt by each individual to control his environment—a typical motivation of individuals who self-injure (Nock 2009, 78)—this mission, in fact, reduces the men's individualism gained through the Fight Club. They now all wear the same clothes and shave their heads as they fulfill orders that Tyler dictates. The Narrator calls them "Space Monkeys" and thus defines them as less than human. That is also the reason why they do not understand that if they make society bleed, they hurt themselves because they are part of society. Here, intrapersonal negative reinforcement can be seen by means of the uniformity Project Mayhem creates, distracting the "Space Monkeys" from any kind of emotion or individual thoughts.

Interpersonal Processes of NSSI in Project Mayhem

The members think that they fled the capitalist system by joining Tyler's organization of Project Mayhem, that this organization is interpersonal and negatively reinforced because it offers an alternative to their previous lives. Ironically, Tyler's organization uses the same methods as the system they tried to escape, that is, a unification of individuals into a following mass. On the other hand, if Project Mayhem is considered an act of self-injury, it can be regarded as a cry for help, which again ties in with NSSI behavior, and attempts to raise awareness to the rottenness of the capitalist system by mirroring the very same system, making it a form of interpersonal positive reinforcement. Project Mayhem incorporates the violence capitalism offers in the form of mental and financial torments and turns it into physical violence. As Žižek (2009, 10) points out, "The notion of objective violence needs to be thoroughly historicized: it took on a new shape with capitalism."

This physical violence is directed at the objective violence, which finds its representatives not just in people, but also in buildings that stand in for culture, such as museums: "The last shot, the tower, all one hundred and ninety-one floors, will slam down on the national museum which is Tyler's real target" (Palahniuk 1996, 14). The latter target plays an important role in so far as Project Mayhem aims at erasing history, at "destroying every scrap of history" (ibid., 12), to build something new, a better society that is freed from old influences. As a consequence, Tyler uses the concept of what the economist Joseph Schumpeter (2000) coined "creative destruction" in 1942. Even though this concept derives from economic studies, it is applicable to literature, in general, and *Fight Club*, in particular. However, with regard to NSSI, the term "creative" seems too abstract and not physical enough, which is why I would like to call the process "constructive destruction."

In *Fight Club*, the cultural memory has to be destroyed in order to construct a new sense of society. In NSSI, a similar phenomenon can be observed. The body—both the individual human body as well as the social body—is destroyed in order to create a sense of selfhood, that is, in order to create an identity which is freed from social constraints. By destroying the social body, society can be rebuilt as a communal unity just like Project Mayhem suggests. The various Fight Clubs that precede Project Mayhem already hint at this destruction of the social body. They are created for the destruction of the individual body, which in turn is supposed to create freedom and individualism.

The members' subsequent involvement in Project Mayhem as an act against capitalism and its oppressive nature is supposed to give the members a purpose in life as a communal group. The members cannot find an identity in the capitalist machine which is regarded as "identity confusion" in NSSI research (Gandhi et al. 2016, 1739). The consequence is alienation from societal (or paternal) norms and a turn toward injuring that very body of the system and by extension, the self as it is still part of the system.

"Late capitalism has commodified the postmodern individual's fears and malaise," argues Tracey Parker (2008, 1). "In late capitalist society, consumers believe in the power of the dollar to the extent that they believe that the act of purchasing will engender solutions for their personal problem" (ibid.). This is exactly what the Narrator tries to do with his IKEA obsession. Yet, in the course of the novel, it becomes clear that materialism is criticized for its confinement. As Irwin (2013, 677) writes, "We are trapped by our possessions—we don't own them, they own us." It is this domination of consumerism that the members of Fight Club want to escape and that the members of Project Mayhem try to fight.

Both Fight Club and Project Mayhem are supposed to give their members a purpose, a meaning in their lives. Even though the motivation for giving life meaning seems plausible, the project is doomed to fail from the beginning because destruction does not lead to construction if communication cannot be guaranteed. In the case of Project Mayhem, there is no communication any more since Tyler dictates everything. Therefore, the members lose their identity, their individuality, and their voice. Thus, after the deeds of destruction, there is no solution offered or discussed for a new beginning. Nobody knows the master plan behind Project Mayhem except for Tyler. Everyone is just a cog in the wheel of the machine. Since Tyler does not share any information with the members nor the Narrator, there is no constructive solution or plan for rebuilding what was destroyed.

The project constructs an idea of masculine power and freedom without actually granting it. Therefore, the project only creates what its name suggests: mayhem. While Fight Club seems to give its members a voice through the individual fights, Project Mayhem takes this voice away through the unification of voices in the form of Tyler Durden. "In Project Mayhem, discourse has truly come to a halt" (Burgess 2012, 275).

INTRAPERSONAL AND INTERPERSONAL COMMUNICATION

Communication is presented in various frames in the novel. On one hand, it can be seen in the concept of museums which attempt to communicate the past to the present so that the future can be constructed. By destroying this form of interpersonal and intra-social communication, an improved societal model is not possible, since the means to improve it—that is, knowledge—is undermined, representing a failure of Freud's "reality principle" (Freud 1930/2010, 29). The latter is to control an individual's development and his or her ability to distinguish between the ego and the outer world, that is, between what is internal or intrapersonal and what is external or interpersonal (relationships, environment) (ibid., 28–29).

The reality principle allows a person to differentiate between intrapersonal communication (thoughts, emotions) and interpersonal communication (in the form of relationships or actual discourse). The Narrator is unable to distinguish between the internal and the external as he externalizes Tyler, even though Tyler is an internal part of him. That is why, as the Narrator, Fight Club, and Project Mayhem show, the destruction of the body does not lead to a construction of the self. Both projects, however, give a sense of life—or rather being alive—as Irwin (2013) explains when he compares and contrasts the support groups to Fight Club:

> Maybe self-improvement is a denial of death, an attempt to put off death, to experience oneself as making something of life, of improving and extending life, whereas self-destruction brings one into close proximity with death. Paradoxically, a brush with death is, as Tyler describes it, "a near-life experience." (678)

Thus, by destroying the self physically and socially, the awareness of existence is foregrounded. It is a thrilling experience, which is described by people who self-injure as "a way of 'transforming' emotional distress into a more manageable physical pain" (Chandler 2012, 444). Similarly, NSSI, as an emotional outlet, can thus also be observed in Fight Club: "While the men may be bruised and scarred physically, they feel better emotionally" (Irwin 2013, 680).

IDENTITY AND NSSI

Identity within Fight Club

Fighters do not only experience NSSI as an emotional outlet; it is also a process of individuation, since the bruises and cuts the men receive during the fights are unique and are thus a sign of individuality and identity. Wounds give the fighters meaning in the form of a physical individual identity. However, even though pain serves as an emotional remedy in Fight Club, the members only experience an illusion of control and masculine identity, but they remain nobodies. The Narrator and the fighters stay anonymous and are thus not able to construct an intrapersonal identity; their identity is only externally visible and can thus be seen as interpersonal.

To take this even further, it is not only the unnamed Narrator's anonymity on an extra- as well as an intra-diegetic level that deny his identity formation, but also his split personality. "The schizophrenic ... has no concrete identity since life events cannot be internalized and put into context" (Parker 2008, 2). While the Narrator had problems of belonging, or rather not belonging, before he met Tyler, he had at least some identity markers through his job and his lifestyle. Tyler, however, takes these away from him completely by promising a fulfilled life through NSSI. This does not give the Narrator an identity of its own, though. Instead, he realizes that he is Tyler Durden.

The failure of establishing an identity can also be observed on another level of failed communication, namely in the rules of Fight Club as well as Project Mayhem. Whereas the first merely forbids verbal discourse and encourages physical communication, the latter intends to extinguish the individual voices of the group members altogether. The first *and* second rules of Fight Club are, "you don't talk about Fight Club" (Palahniuk 1996, 48). Even though it is stated that there should be no discourse *about* Fight Club, within the realms of Fight Club, there is no verbal communication either. The individual's voice is, therefore, transformed into body language by means of the individual fights. Hence, even though the first two rules seem to oppress discourse and aim at silence, they "are intended to encourage communication, since the very existence of Fight Club is spread by word of mouth" (Burgess 2012, 267). The individual voice thus remains powerful to a certain degree because each individual can spread the word.

Identity in Project Mayhem

Fight Club stands in stark contrast to Project Mayhem in so far as the latter unifies the individual voices in the voice of Tyler, which means they are silenced altogether as the first two rules request that "you don't ask questions" (Palahniuk 1996, 131). This negation of communication and the unification process in Project Mayhem is another barrier to create a functioning sense of self. Instead, due to the destruction of the body, the self—that is, each members' individuality—is destroyed and replaced with a homogeneous body of people who have no identity.

Thus, communication among the members is not possible due to their lack of self and personality. They are not able to respond to Tyler's plan in a critical way because they have no longer the freedom to do so. In fact, they are threatened with mutilation if they question Tyler and his project. This mutilation does not fall under the category of self-injury anymore because it is not the individual's choice to be harmed. Thus, while Fight Club encouraged NSSI—each fighter voluntary committed to pain and injuries—Project Mayhem takes freedom of choice away and does not fall under the category of NSSI anymore; this mutilation is not voluntary, but a form of interpersonal punishment. If seen as a group or a social (or rather anti-social) organization, however, mutilation of individual members can be regarded as intra-social.

In addition, communication also fails due to the lack of information the "Space Monkeys" receive. Everyone only has partial knowledge and thus is not able to see the purpose of the project in its entirety. This lack of communicating his intentions puts Tyler in a powerful position, since everyone is dependent on him. He is in control not only of the operation, but also of the body of recruits, or rather, the *bodies* of his recruits. Thus, while Fight Club can still be seen as a special kind of self-injury, Project Mayhem transgresses the boundaries and uses violence against others.

Identity through Death

While the non-suicidal aspect is supposed to be part of Project Mayhem, death still spreads. First, death as murder is included in the chaos and destruction that is caused to society. Death also reaches the inner circles of the club when a club member, Bob, is shot in action. This is the point the Narrator understands what Tyler has created, namely destruction that is all but constructive; it is lethal. The Narrator realizes that this violence against society is in fact suicidal, making it very different from NSSI, and does thus not have the effect of a safety net anymore.

Therefore, again, while Fight Club was focused on NSSI, Project Mayhem seems to shift toward suicide. Instead of feeling alive, Project Mayhem kills in a physical way and in an abstract way, since it takes away one's individuality completely.

Interestingly, once a member dies, his identity is bestowed back upon him, as can be seen in Bob's case. Even though his death is eye-opening to the Narrator, "[t]he epiphany comes with the sight of Bob's corpse" (Burgess 2012, 276), Project Mayhem turns it into a ritual. Members chant Bob's name over and over again in order to give him an identity. However, even though death guarantees identity, the corpse is still caught in a state of nonidentity because the person is gone. The person is thus absent in the presence and present in the absence.

Maurice Blanchot (1989) explains that for the living, death is an imaginary state, a state that is simultaneously possible and impossible in our understanding of it; that is, the concept of death plays with our limitation of knowledge and understanding:

> The cadaverous resemblance haunts us. But its haunting presence is not the unreal visitation of the ideal. What haunts us is something inaccessible from which we cannot extricate ourselves. It is that which cannot be found and therefore cannot be avoided. What no one can grasp is the inescapable. The fixed image knows no repose, and this is above all because it poses nothing, establishes nothing. Its fixity, like that of the corpse, is the position of what says with us because it has no place. (Ibid., 259)

The inaccessibility of death and its fascination by means of near-death experiences is a recurring theme in *Fight Club*. Through risks and pain, death is approached, to be imitated, and to be grasped. But nothing is gained through this because death itself presents nothingness.

Bob's corpse as a physical representation of death is thus reminiscent of Fight Club and Project Mayhem. The members are caught in a condition between feeling alive and dead, which is triggered through pain. Furthermore, they are trapped between the promise of gaining an identity and being individuals, on one hand, and their lack of identity as "Space Monkeys," on the other. However, in the end, they achieve nothing, and they gain nothing. They are still lost in the nihilism of postmodernism. As a consequence, they cannot escape this prison society that Project Mayhem has built for them. Death in its mysterious nothingness suggests the ultimate freedom: that it is not NSSI but suicide that allows an escape.

FREEDOM THROUGH NSSI

The novel's negotiation of how freedom is communicated—that is, if freedom and individuality can only be achieved through death or if it is pain that offers an escape mechanism—is a recurring topic of discussion between the Narrator and Tyler. The latter tries to convince the Narrator that freedom means the rejection of all material goods and rebellion against oppressing forces. These forces are society, on the one hand, and the Narrator's own body, on the other. The bodily oppression can be seen in the Narrator's sleeping problems which stem from a lack of social belonging and a lack of identity.

This lack of identity derives from societal emasculation which results in a longing for male bonding. The latter finds its solution in violence by means of Fight Clubs and, in the Narrator's case, self-injury through schizophrenia. However, while the fights are supposed to reassure the masculine side of the self, the violence against one's own body undermines this attempt. Thus, even though Fight Club and Project Mayhem try to use violence as a masculine force to re-establish a primal masculinity, it is this very use of non-suicidal violence against the self that restricts development of members' masculinity. The reason for this is that they only define masculinity through archaic concepts of the masculine, which highlights their body as the center for gendering.

Interestingly enough, it is Marla Singer, the woman who shows up at the original support groups and the Narrator's/Tyler Durden's love interest, who triggers the Narrator's fear of emasculation and his hallucinations. The entrance of Marla, as a physically healthy, non-decaying woman, prompts the Narrator's need for finding his own masculine identity.

A primal and primitive form of masculinity presents a return to a pre-cultural society in which masculinity (as well as femininity) was clearly defined and gendered. Hence, it is the return to basic instincts that are demanded by Tyler (and indirectly by the Narrator) as well as the members of Project Mayhem. They "destroy corporate urban art and deface luxury cars. These escapades are intended to obliterate the agonizingly mundane trappings of contemporary urban life" (Craine and Aitken 2004, 289). There is a tension here between trapping of the social body and the desires of the individual, or at least, the group around Tyler. The ego cannot balance the opposing forces of the id (basic instincts) and the superego (societal regulations and norms). Violence is the outcome.

This is further manifested by the aforementioned destruction of cultural memory in the form of museums. It is culture that has to be destroyed in order to return to the primal masculine; "we get a sense that either masculinity or culture will cease, and that ultimately the path lies in the transformation of both" (Craine and Aitken 2004, 290). In a postmodern world, this attempt is bound to fail, though, since transformation is based on interpersonal communication, and this is denied in the novel. Instead, intrapersonal suffering is made the point of departure to render an explorative discourse about the crisis of masculinity.

In Palahniuk's *Fight Club*, suffering can thus be discerned on four levels of which Freud determined three (1930, 28). First, there is suffering in the form of bodily decay and physical pain. The second level represents the external suffering caused by societal confinements. The third level discusses the failure of relations with others; this can be seen by means of a lack of communication from the very beginning of the novel. The Narrator does not give his real name in the support groups, which already disables him to establish functioning relationships with others. In addition, the rules of Fight Club make it very clear that communication is not desirable, as discussed earlier.

A fourth level of suffering can be added to be set in relation to postmodern society via the image of the "new" man. The postmodern concept of masculinity does not fit the archaic primal instinct of strength in the primeval hunter who needs to fight to survive and prove his worth in society. Yet, what the men in *Fight Club* are not able to see is that these primal and unified ideas of a clearly gendered society are as oppressing and confining as the fragmented world of postmodernism and thus an unintended self-harm on a social level. What a primal anarchic society is missing is structure and security which allow a certain kind of freedom, but simultaneously deny a peaceful, free, and happy life. Culture and law can at least more or less guarantee security, but only under the condition of a repression of original *ur*-instincts. It is this negotiation between culture and anarchy, between security and chaos, which the Narrator and Tyler engage in and what they represent.

The negotiation takes place on two levels. First, it seems that Tyler and the Narrator discuss these matters on an interpersonal level. However, this interpersonal communication is only a pretense, since Tyler is just a projection of the Narrator's fragmented schizophrenic mind. Thus, it is the second level, the intrapersonal communication that dominates the novel. As "Tyler's voice escalates, the Narrator grows disillusioned, eventually realizing that Tyler is not a separate person but a separate personality" (Burgess 2012, 276). Therefore, the discussion about freedom and masculinity takes place internally and thus shows an individual's inner conflict and struggle with these concepts.

This internalization of conflict leads to an externalization in the form of NSSI since the Narrator is beating himself up and burning himself through Tyler Durden. He not only uses NSSI to communicate with himself by means of Tyler, but he also makes use of it as a way to communicate with others, in particular with the members of Fight Club. This form of communication can once again be linked to Nock's reinforcement processes that maintain NSSI (2009, 79). In the novel as well as in David Fincher's adaptation from 1999, intrapersonal negative reinforcement is thematized by means of the support groups, whereas intrapersonal positive reinforcement is generated by the creation of an imagined alter-ego.

Ironically, negative reinforcement has a positive outcome through its ease of the Narrator's pain, whereas the positive reinforcement has a negative outcome; the latter leads to mayhem. Interpersonal positive reinforcement is mentioned at the very beginning of the story, when the protagonist is seeking help from a doctor. Here again, the outcome is negative since no real help is given. Finally, interpersonal negative reinforcement, that is, the "escape from undesired social situation" (Nock 2009, 79), can be seen in the creation of Fight Club and, on a meta-level, the novel itself as it offers an escape for the reader. In turn, this interpersonal negative reinforcement has a positive outcome by triggering discourse.

Failure of Violence as Communication

With regard to Fight Club and Project Mayhem as interpersonal communication platforms, violence as a means of communication fails. This is why the Narrator ends his internal communication with Tyler through the final violent act of shooting Tyler and, thus, himself. This ultimate act of self-injury does not end in the Narrator's death, but only in his hospitalization. This ending suggests that intrapersonal communication which is based on self-harm and violence, respectively, has to fail because it does not lead to interpersonal relationships.

Burgess (2012, 277) suggests that this "final act of self-destruction and self-abuse is another act of revolutionary liberation" and that the "Narrator regains control over violence, directing it once again toward himself for the sake of liberation and freedom." Consequently, intrapersonal communication has to be identified as such and separated from interpersonal communication in order to be controllable and liberating. Parker (2008) identifies—with regard to David Fincher's adaptation—this failure of change in the very nature of support groups and self-help culture:

> While Fight Club interrogates the "emasculated" world of self-help culture, the film supports the idea that unhappy individuals can latch onto some group whose activities can provide meaning for their lives. Additionally, because self-help culture does not seem to truly solve individual unhappiness nor stimulate change on a societal level, the fact that neither Fight Club nor Project Mayhem result in radical change reflects the reality of self-help culture. (10)

What is left is the gradual learning process of interpersonal communication in order to find individual meaning for one's life.

The surrounding of a mental hospital would, in fact, be a place to learn how to communicate with others and solve problems interpersonally rather than intrapersonally. The novel ends, however, rather ambiguously and before the reader learns about the potential positive influence of the mental institution on the Narrator. Instead, it offers a rather bleak outlook: Tyler's interpersonal communication has been successful insofar as his followers have internalized the violent dogma of Fight Club and Project Mayhem.

A more positive ending is provided by David Fincher's adaptation of *Fight Club*. Here, the Narrator kills his harmful alter-ego by an act of NSSI, that is, by shooting himself in the face, and establishes an interpersonal relationship with Marla Singer. The final scene shows the Narrator and Marla holding hands and watching the destruction of the city. Even though the endings of Palahniuk's novel and Fincher's film are quite different, they both imply that intrapersonal communication based on NSSI has to fail due to the lack of human relationships. After all, throughout the novel, even though we get to know Bob and Marla and some of the followers, "[p]eople are conspicuously absent from Jack's [the Narrator's] life—there is no mention of friends or relatives" (Irwin 2013, 679).

The novel as well as the movie show a rather bleak and lonely world, in which the self is one's greatest enemy, which is why Craine and Aitken (2004, 290) classify *Fight Club* as "a contemporary horror film," in which the bruised and beaten body is the focal point. Parker (2008, 10) confirms this nihilistic horror classification by concluding that "problems are presented, and any solutions that are considered do not engender true social change but instead fool the postmodern subject into thinking that change on the individual level will effectively change their lives."

Even though on a societal level this might hold true, I would argue that on an individual level the transition from intrapersonal to interpersonal communication *can* offer a solution for those who self-injure, as at least Fincher's adaptation suggests. In the realms of NSSI research, the 1992 study by Durand and Carr shows that communication and a time-out from their everyday social environment help people who self-injure to open up and externalize their feelings through interpersonal communication instead of through self-harm (Hastings and Noone 2005, 336). This can also be observed in *Fight Club* as the Narrator takes a form of time-out by abandoning the societal conformities and living an alternate life. This form is not sustainable, but interpersonal communication is or might be.

Relationships eventually present what Irwin calls "creative replacement" which follows after destruction in order to fill life with meaning (cf. Irwin 682). Gandhi et al. (2016) confirm that "communication may also reduce interpersonal alienation" (1743). It is thus only in non-violent interpersonal relationships that individuality and identity can be found, which makes *Fight Club*, despite its emphasis on masculinity, a romance novel in disguise. Early on in the novel, the Narrator acknowledges that "[w]ithout Marla, Tyler would have nothing" (Palahniuk 1996, 14) and by extension, the Narrator would have nothing.

As in many romances, it is the absence of interpersonal communication that leads to conflict. Thus, in order to establish relationships, a sense of identity has to be established. This, in turn, can only be achieved by fighting the self in order to conquer the self and survive to finally open up to others through *non*-violent communication. As the endings of both the novel and the film suggest, only when the self-injury stops, the healing can begin and interpersonal communication and thus relationships are possible.

BIBLIOGRAPHY

Adler, Patricia A., and Peter Adler. *The Tender Cut: Inside the Hidden World of Self-Injury*. New York: New York University Press, 2011.

Anderson, Emily R. "Telling Stories: Unreliable Discourse, Fight Club, and the Cinematic Narrator." *Journal of Narrative Theory* 40, no. 1 (2010): 80–107.

Bareiss, Warren. "Adolescent Daughters and Ritual Abjection: Narrative Analysis of Self-Injury in Four US Films." *Journal of Medical Humanities* 38, no. 3 (2017): 319–337.

Blanchot, Maurice. *The Space of Literature*. Translated by Ann Smock. Lincoln, London: University of Nebraska Press, 1989.

Burgess, Olivia. "Revolutionary Bodies in Chuck Palahniuk's *Fight Club*." *Utopian Studies* 23, no. 1 (2012): 263–280.

Chandler, Amy. "Self-Injury as Embodied Emotion Work: Managing Rationality, Emotions and Bodies." *Sociology* 46, no. 3 (2012): 442–457.

Craine, James, and Stuart Aitken. "Street Fighting: Placing the Crisis of Masculinity in David Fincher's Fight Club." *GeoJournal* 59, no. 4 (2004): 289–296.

Fincher, David, dir. *Fight Club*. 20th Century Fox, 1999.

Freud, Sigmund. *Civilization and Its Discontent 1930*. Mansfield Centre, CT: Martino Publishing, 2010.

Gandhi, Amarendra, Laurence Claes, Guy Bosmans, Imke Baetens, Tom F. Wilderjans, Shubhada Maitra, Glenn Kiekens, and Koen Luyckx. "Non-Suicidal Self-Injury and Adolescents Attachment with Peers and Mother: The Mediating Role of Identity Synthesis and Confusion." *Journal of Child and Family Studies* 25, no. 6 (2016): 1735–1745.

Gilman, Sander L. "From Psychiatric Symptom to Diagnostic Category: Self-Harm from the Victorians to DSM-5." *History of Psychiatry* 24, no. 2 (2013): 148–165.

Giroux, Henry A. "Private Satisfactions and Public Disorders: *Fight Club*, Patriarchy, and the Politics of Masculine Violence." *JAC* 21, no. 1 (2001): 1–31.

Hastings, Richard P., and Stephen J. Noone. "Self-Injurious Behavior and Functional Analysis: Ethics and Evidence." *Education and Training in Developmental Disabilities* 40, no. 4 (2005): 335–342.

Hustvedt, Siri. "Three Emotional Stories: Reflections on Memory, the Imagination, Narrative, and the Self." *Neuropsychoanalysis* 13, no. 2 (2011): 187–196.

Irwin, William. "Fight Club, Self-Definition, and the Fragility of Authenticity." *Revista Portuguesa de Filosofia* 69, no. 3/4 (2013): 673–684.

Kavadlo, Jesse. "The Fiction of Self-Destruction: Chuck Palahniuk, Closet Moralist." In *You Do Not Talk About Fight Club*, edited by Read Mercer Schuchardt, 13–33. Dallas, TX: BenBella Books, 2008.

Millard, Chris. "Making the Cut: The Production of 'Self-Harm' in Post-1945 Anglo-Saxon Psychiatry." *History of the Human Sciences* 26, no. 2 (2013): 126–150.

Nock, Matthew K. "Why Do People Hurt Themselves? New Insights into the Nature and Function of Self-Injury." *Current Directions in Psychological Science* 18, no. 2 (2009): 78–83.

Palahniuk, Chuck. *Fight Club 1996*. London: Vintage Books, 2006.

Parker, Tracey K. "Do I Lie to Myself to Be Happy?: Self-Help Culture and Fragmentation in Postmodern Film." *Interdisciplinary Literary Studies* 10, no. 1 (2008): 1–5.

Schumpeter, Joseph. *Capitalism, Socialism and Democracy*. London: Routledge, 2000.

Shedden, David. "New Media Timeline (1996)." *Poynter* (2004). 17 February 2020. https://www.poynter.org/archive/2004/new-media-timeline-1996/.

Žižek, Slavoj. *Violence*. London: Profile Books, 2009.

Chapter 9

A Systematic Review of Media Use and Non-Suicidal Self-Injury Behaviors

Shuang Liu and Yanni Ma

INTRODUCTION

Self-injury occurs when someone intentionally and repeatedly harms themselves in a way that is not intended to be suicidal. Non-suicidal self-injury (NSSI) is the second leading cause of death for people aged fifteen to nineteen years old (Centers for Disease Control and Prevention 2017). Studies have found that seventeen percent to thirty-five percent college students and twenty-three percent of adolescents have engaged in NSSI at some point in their lives (e.g., Muehlenkamp and Gutierrez 2007; Whitlock et al. 2006). In addition, mental health providers have also acknowledged the increased prevalence of NSSI over time, making it a significant concern for public health and social care practice.

Portrayals of self-injury behaviors appear in a variety of media formats including books, movies, music videos, online forums, and social media. Looking at movies, TV shows, and music in the English language, researchers have identified an increase in the amount of self-injury depictions since 2000, with ten times more explicit references to self-injury between 2000 to 2005, compared to prior to the 1990s (Whitlock et al. 2009). More importantly, research found that close to half (43.6%) of the adolescents and young adults reported that media exposure had an impact on their NSSI behaviors (Heath et al. 2008). The role of media, especially social media, on NSSI has garnered increasing attention from health practitioners and researchers.

Despite a growing body of literature from public health examining media use and deliberate self-harm acts (e.g., Cavazos-Rehg et al. 2017; Seko and

Lewis 2018), the association remains unclear between media consumption habits and self-injury among adolescents and young adults from communication perspectives.

There is extensive research in communication on how media use can influence an individual's beliefs, knowledge, attitudes, and behaviors when it comes to health-related issues. One of the most prominent communication theoretical frameworks explaining the effect of media consumption is social cognitive theory. Social cognitive theory posits that people often acquire new behaviors by observing and modeling others around them, and as such, they can learn vicariously by watching others in the media, such as celebrities, movie characters, and so forth (Bandura 1986). According to social cognitive theory, viewers may change their attitudes and behaviors based on whether a certain behavior is being rewarded or punished in the media portrayal.

A strategic communication strategy called "entertainment education" is derived from social cognitive theory. The use of entertainment education in the media has been found to be effective in health-related messages and interventions in influencing people's attitudes, knowledge, beliefs, and behaviors such as sexual health and alcohol consumption. For example, *Friends* (a popular American sitcom television series aired from 1994 to 2004) featured an episode in which the male characters discuss the use of condoms. This episode deliberately incorporated a message about the success rate of condoms. Not long after the episode aired, a group of researchers conducted a telephone survey of 506 adolescents aged twelve to seventeen years old who had been regular viewers of the show the previous year (Collins et al. 2003). The survey questions include recall of the condom-efficacy message, beliefs about condoms, self-reported change in condom knowledge, and discussions of condom efficacy with parents. The study found that entertainment program, if used strategically, can serve as a sex educator to increase knowledge regarding sexual health as well as facilitate conversations on health-related topics between adolescents and their parents.

In a similar vein, a study found that college students who watched the episode of the TV show *ER* where an anti-alcohol message was shown, reported less positive attitudes and lower behavioral intentions to binge drink than those who did not see the message (Kim et al. 2014).

While researchers and health practitioners have applied communication theories in the development and assessment of various health care interventions, inquiry of the theoretical processes through which media consumption influence NSSI has been largely lacking. As NSSI is rapidly growing in public awareness and becoming a serious public health concern, it is vital to understand the mechanisms through which media use influences attitudes and behaviors regarding NSSI. Furthermore, researchers have suggested using theory guided messages and techniques to develop health campaigns as to practice effective interventions (Noar and Mehrotra 2011). No systematic literature review to date has focused on media use and self-harm among adolescents and young adults. Therefore, the current chapter aims to fill this gap and review the existing literatures in relation to media use on NSSI behaviors. Specifically, this systematic review will answer the following research questions:

RQ 1: What is the linkage between self-injury and media use found in the current research?
RQ 2: Is there any communication theory used in the studies? If so, what is the theory?

Finally, this chapter will also identify recommendations for future research and interventions.

RESEARCH METHOD

With an ever-growing body of empirical research being published in communication and public health, reviews summarizing the findings of various studies and interventions can offer an efficient look at a certain topic and provide the "bottom line about what works and what doesn't" (Uman 2011, 57). Systematic reviews typically involve a comprehensive search strategy proposed by the author a priori. The author then identifies and selects all the studies that fit certain inclusion and exclusion criteria related to the research questions/hypotheses on a particular topic. A systematic review is informative in this case because it can illustrate the current state of research in the relationship between self-injury and media consumption, and the use of theory in the published studies, thus providing an evidence-based discussion on what is existing and needed in this line of inquiry as well as what clinicians and health care intervention developers in this field can do to combat NSSI.

IDENTIFICATION OF STUDIES

Two authors conducted an extensive search for relevant articles published in English-language peer-reviewed journals published before November 2018. Databases including PsychINFO, Medline, Cumulative Index of Nursing and Allied Health Literature, Academic Search Complete, and Communication and Mass Media Complete using the terms self-injur* or self-harm and media or communication were searched. The initial search yielded 599 articles. After duplicates were removed, 482 articles were archived in an Endnote (ver. 7.8) database.

All the articles that were considered for inclusion in this systematic review met the following criteria:

1. Studies had to be original research and could not be secondary data analysis.
2. Studies had to be published in peer-reviewed journals and books.

One researcher reviewed the search results and selected papers that met the inclusion criteria for the study. Protocol was created, and another researcher coded a subset of the articles. Articles were screened in several stages using explicit inclusion criteria (see figure 9.1). First, the citations were reviewed to judge their eligibility for the systematic review. Abstracts were evaluated and ineligible articles were excluded ($n = 387$). Abstracts of the remaining articles ($n = 95$) were further evaluated and studies that were not original studies (i.e., data collection and analysis) were excluded. Abstracts that did not explicitly indicate how the researchers collected data were set aside to determine each study's eligibility through a review of the methods section of the article.

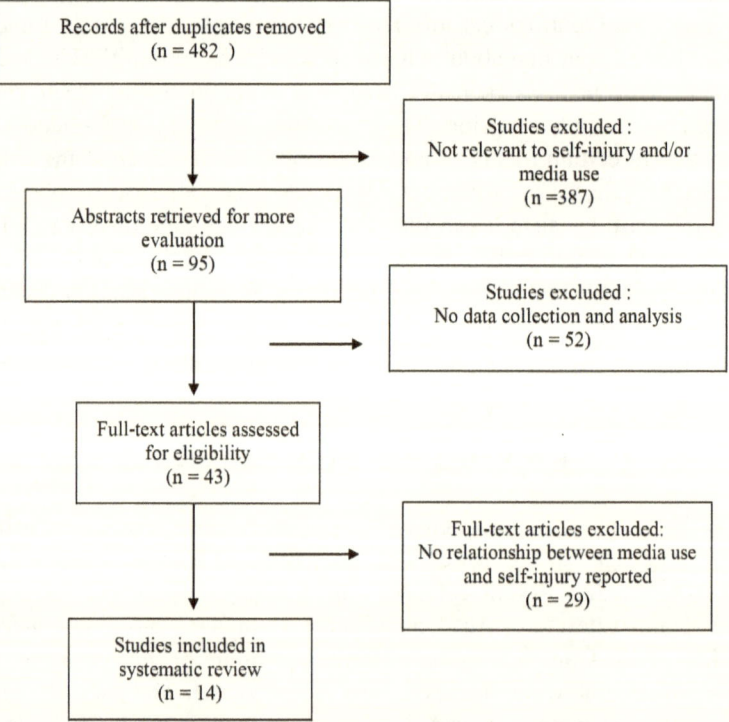

Figure 9.1 Summary of Selection Process. *Source:* Author Created.

Full-text copies of the remaining forty-three potentially relevant articles were examined more closely. Out of the forty-three articles, only fourteen clearly reported media consumption and self-injury. Finally, backward searching (reviewing the reference lists of the articles for any missed studies) and forward searching (checking the articles that had cited the articles that had been selected for inclusion) were conducted to ensure no additional eligible studies were missed from the search.

ARTICLE CODING

The authors coded the eligible studies independently on a number of variables related to the research questions including study design, theoretical framework, participants, methodology, and so forth. A subset of articles ($n = 5$) were coded by the second author to make sure coding was consistent (intercoder reliability = eighty-five percent). Operational definitions were discussed prior to the coding process to ensure the categorization was consistently applied throughout the process.

RESULTS

Although a total number of forty-three articles received full-text review, only fourteen studies that clearly reported the use of media and NSSI behaviors were selected for this systematic review. All of the studies used qualitative research methods (e.g., in-depth interview, textual analysis) ($n = 14$). For example, one study used transcripts extracted from an online discussion forum to analyze the conversations between health care professionals and participants who engage in self-injury (Smithson et al. 2011). The sample of the studies was mainly adolescents (aged fourteen to seventeen years old) ($n = 9$) and young adults (aged eighteen to twenty-two years old) ($n = 5$). As for the type of media platform, all of the studies focused on the Internet. Specifically, three studies looked at online forums and message boards, and all the other studies looked at social media, including Instagram ($n = 3$), Tumblr ($n = 4$), Twitter ($n = 2$), Youtube ($n = 1$), and a combination of Twitter, Instagram, and Tumblr ($n = 1$).

The first research question asked whether and how the current research investigated the linkage between media consumption and NSSI behaviors. The results showed that only one study has reported the relationship between media use habits and self-harm related attitudes and behaviors (Hilton 2016). The study conducted in the UK used inductive thematic analysis to analyze 362 Twitter messages and found that even though Twitter may be considered a source of understanding and provides a sense of community for people who engage in self-harm, through continued usage, such support seems to also contribute to the normalization of self-harm and, in turn, perpetuate the behavior of the users. None of the other studies selected in the review reported any association between media use habits and NSSI behaviors.

The second research question dealt with how communication theory is applied in the current research concerning media use and self-injury behaviors. Out of all the studies reviewed, only one study was conducted in the context of a theory. Brown et al. (2018) used the self-injury pictures downloaded from Instagram during four weeks in 2016 using the hashtag #cutting to investigate the association between pictures and comments and the trends of posting behaviors. The researchers found that social reinforcement played an important role in users posting more pictures of severe wounds, as they often led to greater responses and more comments.

DISCUSSION

NSSI has become one of the most concerning health and social issues concerning adolescents and young adults. With the growing interest in self-harm acts in the media, especially the possibility of perpetuating such acts in social media, there is a crucial need for investigating the relationship between media use and self-injury behaviors.

The current chapter used a systematic review to examine how the current research in the field of communication studied the effect of media use on NSSI as well as the theoretical processes through which media influence such behaviors. The findings suggested that most research was interested in the use of social media (e.g., Twitter, Tumblr, Instagram) to analyze the communication among people who engage in self-injury. This could be due to the popularity of social media among adolescents and young adults and the privacy that social media channels afford the users. It is interesting that all the studies used either adolescents or young adults as their study sample which echoes researchers' and health professionals' concerns for this population. In addition, all of the studies used qualitative research methods. Even though qualitative inquiry can provide an in-depth and nuanced look into the issue, more quantitative research is needed to compliment the investigation and inform effective interventions by examining the contributing variables and the significant relationships between media use and self-injury.

Even though research shows that exposure to media portrayals of self-harm acts has an impact on how viewers conduct such behaviors (Heath et al. 2008), the current review shows that, out of fourteen reviewed articles, only one reported how media consumption (e.g., Twitter) can potentially lead to more self-injury (Hilton 2016). This finding shows that the effect of media consumption—mass media and social media—on people who self-injure versus those who don't self-injure is understudied, even though decades of communication research shows that mass media can have tremendous impact on people's perceptions, knowledge, attitudes, and behaviors in various health issues. Furthermore, the lack of research on the linkage between the use of social media and self-injury attitudes and behaviors is also problematic, as social media websites play such an important part in adolescents' and young adults' daily lives. Therefore, it is imperative for more investigation into how media use habits can positively or negatively influence adolescents' beliefs, attitudes, and behaviors.

The current review also found that there is a lack of the use of theory guiding the research. This is concerning, as some researchers have argued the importance of using communication theory to explain individuals' health behaviors, inform future research, and create effective campaigns to combat this issue (Noar and Mehrotra 2011). As previous studies have demonstrated, communication theories, such as social cognitive theory, can be used to explain the processes through which media impact self-injury attitudes and behaviors. Theories can also be used to guide efficient evidence-based intervention efforts to help combat such health issues.

This line of research indicates that media consumption—for example, social media—generally has a negative impact on adolescents and young adults' self-injury behaviors, as they could normalize the behaviors and serve as a convenient platform to foster and encourage the maintenance of self-injury behaviors. Health interventions could focus on tracking the self-injury content, and providing more positive feedback for the victims when they are not ready to share their stories. It is more important to be aware of the reactance among young people sharing their experiences and accept clinical treatment. Because these young people have their own communities, interventions could also be developed to customize to the specific community. For instance, practitioners could use more "coded" languages than frequently being used within the community.

LIMITATIONS AND FUTURE DIRECTIONS

The current study was a narrative systematic review and, therefore, could not provide a quantitative look into and precise estimates of the effect sizes of the reviewed studies. However, the fact that the researchers did a thorough and systematic search of the literature and only found limited numbers of studies that meet the inclusion criteria is an indication of how underdeveloped the literature is around this topic. Future research is needed to evaluate the effect sizes when there is a much larger body of evidence in this field. In addition, future investigation could use more quantitative approaches to examine whether consuming information including images and texts on self-injury is associated with attitudinal and behavioral change. For instance, more could be done related to what specific messages or content could affect individuals' normalization of self-injury, and why.

Further, NSSI and health communication scholars can also look at the interactions between young people on the topic or self-injury. Specifically, it will be interesting to look at how they respond to self-injury content, and whether the person who posts self-injury information is open to conversations with other social media users.

CONCLUSIONS

In light of the increasing concern regarding media consumption and self-injury among adolescents and young adults, the current study used a systematic review to examine how the current research has been conducted to understand the relationship and the theoretical processes through with media influence self-injury behaviors. The findings revealed that there is a lack of research on how media consumption can contribute to self-injury behaviors. In addition, the current research in this area is not guided by communication theory. More quantitative and long-term investigation need to be conducted to identify the linkage between media consumption and self-injury behaviors. There is also dire need for the development of theory-grounded health communication campaigns.

REFERENCES

Bandura, Albert. *Social Foundations of Thought and Action: A Social Sognitive Theory*. Upper Saddle River, NJ: Prentice-Hall, Inc., 1986.

Brown, R. C., T. Fischer, A. D. Goldwich, F. Keller, R. Young, and P. L. Plener. "#Cutting: Non-Suicidal Self-Injury (NSSI) on Instagram." *Psychological Medicine* 48 (2017): 337–346. doi:10.1017/s0033291717001751

Cavazos-Rehg, Patricia A., Melissa J. Krauss, Shaina J. Sowles, Sarah Connolly, Carlos Rosas, Meghana Bharadwaj, Richard Grucza, and Laura J. Bierut. "An Analysis of Depression, Self-Harm, and Suicidal Ideation Content on Tumblr." *Crisis* 38, no. 1 (2017): 44–52. doi:10.1027/0227-5910/a000409

Centers for Disease Control and Prevention. *Suicide and Self-Inflicted Injury*, 2017. Retrieved from https://www.cdc.gov/nchs/fastats/suicide.htm

Collins, Rebecca L., Marc N. Elliott, Sandra H. Berry, David E. Kanouse, and Sarah B. Hunter. "Entertainment Television as a Healthy Sex Educator: The Impact of

Condom-Efficacy Information in an Episode of *Friends.*" *Pediatrics* 112, no. 5 (2003): 1115–1121.

Heath, Nancy L., Kristin Schaub, Shareen Holly, and Mary K. Nixon. "Self-Injury Today: Review of Population and Clinical Studies in Adolescents." In *Self-Injury in Youth: The Essential Guide to Assessment and Intervention,* edited by Mary K. Nixon and Nancy L. Heath, 9–28. New York, NY: Routledge, 2008.

Hilton, C. "Unveiling Self-Harm Behaviour: What Can Social Media Site Twitter Tell Us About Self-Harm? A Qualitative Exploration." *Journal of Clinical Nursing* 26 (2017): 1690–1704. doi:10.1111/jocn.13575

Kim, Kyongseok, Mina Lee, and Wendy Macias. "An Alcohol Message Beneath the Surface of ER: How Implicit Memory Influences Viewers' Health Attitudes and Intentions Using Entertainment-Education." *Journal of Health Communication* 19 (2014): 876–892.

Muehlenkamp, Jennifer J., and Peter M. Gutierrez. "Risk for Suicide Attempts Among Adolescents Who Engage in Non-Suicidal Self-Injury." *Archives of Suicide Research* 11, no. 1 (2007): 69–82. doi:10.1080/13811110600992902

Noar, Seth M., and Purnima Mehrotra. "Toward a New Methodological Paradigm for Testing Theories of Health Behavior and Health Behavior Change: Patient Education and Counseling." *Patient Education and Counseling* 82, no. 3 (2011): 468–474. doi:10.1016/j.pec.2010.11.016

Seko, Yukari, and Stephen P. Lewis. "The Self—Harmed, Visualized, and Reblogged: Remaking of Self-Injury Narratives on Tumblr." *New Media & Society* 20, no. 1 (2016): 180–198. doi:10.1177/1461444816660783

Smithson, Janet, Siobhan Sharkey, Elaine Hewis, Ray Jones, Tobit Emmens, Tamsin Ford, and Christabel Owens. "Problem Presentation and Responses on an Online Forum for Young People Who Self-Harm." *Discourse Studies* 13, no. 4 (2011): 487–501. doi:10.1177/1461445611403356

Uman, Lindsay S. "Systematic Reviews and Meta-Analyses." *Journal of the Canadian Academy of Child and Adolescent Psychiatry* 20, no. 1 (2011): 57–59.

Whitlock, Janis, Amanda Purington, and Marina Gershkovich. "Media, the Internet, and Nonsuicidal Self-Injury." In *Understanding Nonsuicidal Self-Injury: Origins, Assessment, and Treatment,* edited by Matthew K. Nock, 139–155. Washington, DC: American Psychological Association, 2009.

Whitlock, Janis, Greg Eells, Nina Cummings, and Amanda Purington. "Nonsuicidal Self-Injury in College Populations: Mental Health Provider Assessment of Prevalence and Need." *Journal of College Student Psychotherapy* 23, no. 3 (2009): 172–183. doi:1080/87568220902794366

Whitlock, Janis, John Eckenrode, and Daniel Silverman. "Self-Injurious Behaviors in a College Population." *Pediatrics* 117, no. 6 (2006): 1939–1948. doi:10.1542/peds.2005-2543

Chapter 10

The End (a.k.a The Beginning)

Application of Buddhist Principles in Communicating With, About, and Through Self-Harm

Warren J. Bareiss

During the final months of editing this book, when the end seemed very far away, I was comforted by a short song written and recorded by Donovan called "There is a Mountain." There is one line that I particularly like about a caterpillar becoming a butterfly. Unfortunately, copyright law forbids me from telling you any of the lyrics, but you can find them in about thirty seconds online.

I found myself singing "There is a Mountain" over and over as I went about my work for nearly three months. East and West meet in this little tune so indicative of 1960s countercultural wonder, joy, and optimism. The song was apparently inspired by the Buddhist scholar, Qingyuan Weixin, who is credited with saying:

> Before I had studied Ch'an [Zen[1]] for thirty years, I saw mountains as mountains, and rivers as rivers. When I arrived at a more intimate knowledge, I came to the point where I saw that mountains are not mountains, and rivers are not rivers. But now that I have got its very substance, I am at rest. For it's just that I see mountains once again as mountains, and rivers once again as rivers. (Lopez 2008)

Donovan's song (and Qingyuan Weixin's words) tell me that nothing is permanent except for change. Also, perception is imperfect, and identities are in constant flow. I often thought that if I could gift a song to people whose stories are reflected in these chapters, that would be the one.

When I first started this project two years ago, I happened to take my son, who was about twelve years old at the time, to a doctor for a reason that I now forget. Chatting with the pediatrician, I thought that he would be able to give me unique insight into non-suicidal self-injury (NSSI), since self-injury is so often associated with young people. He told me that, from what he saw, girls were prone to what we would normally consider NSSI—most often, cutting. "Boys," and here, he included adolescents, "do other things like drive too fast." That conversation bothered me throughout the process of putting this book together, causing me some degree of cognitive dissonance. How can driving too fast be NSSI? It doesn't fit the model available in the scholarship, yet I couldn't get it out of my mind right up until writing this conclusion. Working through this last chapter in the book, I think I understand.

Authors whose work I was fortunate to collect in this book have examined NSSI in many communicative contexts: within the individual (chapters 3 and 5), among family members (chapter 4), amid healthcare settings (chapters 1 and 2), in scholarship (chapter 9), and among media representations (chapters 6–8). Throughout the book, authors have been consistent in how they define NSSI, and we have seen general agreement on the functionality of NSSI among those who engage in it. This functionality, as was demonstrated in multiple chapters, serves to provide people who self-injure temporary emotional relief from ongoing life stressors and/or a sense of control over their lives amid chaotic circumstances.

Throughout this book, we have seen a mix of suggested and empirically supported methods for engaging with patients in immediate crisis and in ongoing therapy such as improving supportive sibling communication (chapter 4), re-routing NSSI to more productive stress responses (chapter 5), helping clients develop language skills to express their internal states (chapter 2), and teaching patients ways to handle stress (chapter 1). These skills are presented as possible strategies in working with individual patients, but I am left with a question that moves beyond case-by-case treatment: What are we to do about NSSI as a widespread *social pattern* beyond day-to-day engagement with patients, clients, friends, and family?

I write this conclusion in the midst of the COVID-19 pandemic. My family and I have hardly left our neighborhood in four months. "Social distancing" has taken me away from colleagues, friends, and students, but, surprisingly, has also afforded me time to think, build a garden, and catch up on some reading. For many years, I have had the habit of purchasing books about Buddhism and meditation and never actually reading past the first few pages. I thought that Buddhism might offer me some sense of purpose and peace in a world filled with conflict and stress, but until the past few months, I didn't have time to really engage with them.

Paging through a couple of the books over the years, I understood the basic premises of Buddhism exemplified in the Four Noble Truths: Life is conditioned by suffering. Suffering is caused by craving. Suffering can be ended. Suffering can be ended by following the Eightfold Path. And that's where I inevitably stopped reading. The Eightfold Path requires commitment, and commitment requires time.

The pandemic gave me the time that I needed. I began with *How to Sit* by renowned Zen writer and teacher, Thich Nhat Hanh (2019). As I read and learned rudimentary meditation skills, it occurred to me that Buddhist philosophy offered some concepts that could be useful in communicating with clients, patients, friends, family, colleagues, and the general public about ways to *embrace* NSSI rather than to combat it. By that, I don't mean that I think that NSSI is a good thing that we should preserve, but rather, maybe we should try to bring it out of the shadows and reconsider its associated stigma.

In writing these concluding thoughts, in no way do I want to present myself as an expert in Buddhism, nor is my attempt to sell Buddhism to my readers. Rather, I am inspired by Elisa Aaltola's (2019) insightful article reframing how we can think about disabilities. Contrasting typical Western thinking with Zen Buddhist philosophy, Aaltola writes

> In the context of disability, the Zen Buddhist approach would urge one to cease all efforts to render disability into a permanent "essence" that defines oneself, and similarly it would persuade one to stop making it "meaningful" via, for instance, narratives that underline the sort of epistemic transformation that seeks truthful permanence. Moreover, efforts to fully and potentially govern one's condition and identity emerge as unproductive and merely lead to more anguish. From the perspective of Zen Buddhist thinking, instead of identity reclamations, disabled individuals would benefit from letting go of the attachment to given, fixed identities and stories constructing them. (p. 238)

While Aaltola's specific application is toward disability studies, I found her argument refreshingly useful in thinking about NSSI.

I am not the first to link Buddhism and NSSI. Numerous books, chapters, and articles—including chapter 1 of this book—apply the notion of "mindfulness" to the study and treatment of NSSI, almost always using Marsha Linehan's (Linehan 1993a, 1993b; Dimeff and Linehan 2001) application of the term with respect to dialectical behavior therapy (DBT) (see, for example, Muehlenkamp 2006; Van Gelder 2010). "Mindfulness" is a meditative technique wherein the person is fully aware in the moment, accepting and recognizing thoughts and emotions as they arise *as* thoughts and emotions (see, for example, Shapiro 2009). Application and discussion of mindfulness in psychological literature is vast and worthy of further reading (see, for example, Robins 2002). Other references to other existential aspects of Buddhist philosophy in NSSI scholarship are harder to come by and still quite tenuous (see, for example, Jiang et al. 2017).

As a newcomer to Buddhism, it would be impertinent of me to present this concluding chapter as anything more than food for thought, that is, some suggestions for moving forward based upon a few concepts that I have uncovered in my informal study. At the same time, as I plunge into new territory, I can't help but feel an excitement for exploration and learning about NSSI that I have not felt in a long time. In Zen Buddhism, my eagerness and wonder in the newness of this topic are referred to as "the beginner's mind" (see Suzuki 1970). Perhaps my beginner's exploration might inspire similar, excitement, curiosity, and openness among other scholars and healthcare providers. By that, I mean both scholars and clinicians who are experts in NSSI, but know little or nothing about Buddhism, as well as those who are already skilled in Eastern philosophy, but know nothing of NSSI. Now, there is an idea for a conference that I would like to attend!

In the following few pages, my goal is to suggest how we might develop our means of communicating about the nature of NSSI and what we can do about it using four concepts common in Buddhist philosophy: impermanence, compassion, suffering, and mindfulness. The concepts are drawn from three basic principles of Buddhist thinking (see Thera 1987/1993): Nothing is permanent, suffering is a basic fact of life, and the concept of self is illusory. These three principles can be challenging to scholars and clinicians accustomed to Western style of thinking, but I will try to demonstrate their potential practicality with respect to NSSI. Writing at a very general level, I will dispense with the usual storm of references and rather guide readers to my go-to introductory text, *An Introduction to the Buddha and His Teachings* (Bercholz and Kohn 1993) for further reading.

As mentioned above, I write this conclusion from my home in South Carolina approximately five months into the COVID-19 pandemic. In my suburban neighborhood, I see people going about their business as if nothing unusual is happening. Neighbors chat among themselves pretty much as always without even the protection of social distancing. Many of my neighbors—like millions of their fellow countrywomen and countrymen—live in denial about the serious danger of contagion, with a "second wave" almost certainly on the horizon.

Based upon what I see in the news, much of that denial is associated with perceptions about loss of freedom. Many people don't like to be told to wear masks or to stay at home. This is a control issue. Who has the power to control what we wear and where we go? And at a deeper level, who has the power to mandate that we inconvenience ourselves for the protection of others?

Desire for control of the world around is one side of the proverbial coin, and freedom to do as we wish is the other. Both sides are intimately realized through control of one's body and, conversely, through the control of other people's bodies. Humans go to great lengths to make this point to themselves and others. Fashions of all types including apparel, body art, and hairstyles are expressions of autonomy pertaining to the body. Similarly, control of others often means enacting restrictions on all those forms of expression, not to mention more structurally formalized institutions such as prison and legal restrictions on what we can and can't do with our bodies. Indeed, sometimes people's bodies are the only channels open for expressing any form of control over their lives.

As we have seen throughout this book, people who self-injure also seek control, and again, the body is the nexus of behavior, communication, and meaning. Control might pertain to perceived sense of self, relationships with others, or the general social environment. In one way or another, people who self-injure turn to cutting, burning, banging, and other forms of NSSI because it gives them a sense, however temporary, of self-efficacy (see chapter 2, for example). The *moment* of self-injury brings relief, but the *process* of self-injury becomes one of self-empowerment. The action might be followed by regret (as in chapter 7), but the cycle goes round and round as a short-term defense mechanism wherein the idealized self battles internal and external conflicts.

Multiple chapters here have described how responses among healthcare providers and scholars encourage people who practice NSSI to concentrate on constructing the self in more productive ways—through storytelling, cognitive behavioral therapy, writing diaries, and so on (e.g., chapters 3–5). And we have seen some evidence that emphasis on reinforcing self-identity has positive effect on patients' well-being and desire to self-injure (chapters 1 and 2).

Emphasis on oneself is indicative of Western perceptions of identity and individualism. It is an especially powerful American ideal with a variety of expressions to match: "stand on your own two feet," for example, and the value attributed to "rugged individualism." On the other hand, emphasis on the self carries some risk, especially regarding blame. If one doesn't succeed in reaching their goals, who is to blame but oneself? And this brings us back to control. If the focus is on oneself to make everything just right, how often can a person fully succeed in a complex world with infinite possibilities that can't be controlled?

Aaltola (2019) argues that control as emphasized in Western culture runs contrary to Zen Buddhist philosophy because control is a form of desire or clinging to illusory perceptions of a permanent reality. This clinging can only lead to despair because the things that we perceive as permanent are, in reality, always changing. Therefore, what we think of as this or that is a fantasy of permanence projected onto fluidity. We can never really control anything because things don't exist as we perceive them, and for that matter, neither do we. Desire thus leads to perpetual suffering in the longing for that which we cannot have.

Furthermore, given the fluid nature and impermanence of everything, attempts to define anything are doomed to failure because distinctions between one thing and another are only a matter of momentary convenience. Indeed, from the start of putting this book together, I ran into this very problem as mentioned above while discussing NSSI with my son's pediatrician. What is NSSI, really? Multiple chapters in this book use the same definition, but in reality, that definition has very leaky seams. If NSSI is deliberate harming of one's body without suicidal intent, what about people who sometimes self-injure in that way *and* sometimes attempt suicide? Or, if we only include people who don't attempt suicide, how do we classify smokers who know that cigarettes could kill them? What about binge drinkers? Or "workaholics?"

Aaltola (2019) posits that rather than encourage people with disabilities to focus on their identities as "disabled" (assuming we could ever agree on a definition), would it not be at least be equally beneficial to emphasize the *experience of* being disabled as a range of possibilities? Rather than rejecting pain, discomfort, inconvenience, and so forth, we can embrace it. Rather than separating disabled from abled, such an approach would integrate people with disabilities into a continuity of human experience united by varying degrees of universal suffering. Such an approach, Aaltola argues, not only emphasizes the humanness of disabilities, but directs attention outward to pain shared by everyone in some way or another. The emphasis is not on the unique circumstances of the individual, but rather, the shared suffering of humanity. It's about connection rather than separation and about commonality rather than difference.

One of the causes of anxiety among people who self-injure is that the act of NSSI itself is stigmatized. Therefore, it is easy to assume that one is somehow aberrant if she or he self-harms. This can lead to feelings of guilt and isolation and then back to self-injury.

What if we were to widen the definition of NSSI to *all* forms of deliberate self-harm without suicidal intent so as to include drinking too much alcohol, smoking, using recreational drugs, overworking, putting oneself into stressful situations, having risky sex, drinking too much caffeine, eating fatty foods, over-stressing, continuously ruminating about unhappy circumstances, falling in love with the wrong people over and over, and being too outspoken in faculty meetings? The list could be endless. Given this expanded definition, doesn't everyone self-injure? If we all do it, it can't be aberrant. Practicing self-injury is, from this perspective, part of the human condition.

Were we to approach NSSI with a much broader, dynamic perspective, patients who engage in what we have traditionally thought of as NSSI would not be constructed as members of a class unto themselves. They are just people doing what people often do in many different ways. If one person self-injures with a razor blade and another by being a workaholic, how are they really different? Thinking of NSSI in this way de-stigmatizes the behavior, making it more likely that people who self-injure will be more comfortable communicating with friends, family members, and healthcare providers about their behaviors. Ideally, that communication will lead to further communication about the root causes of NSSI and, perhaps, resolution of mitigating external factors.

Assuming that suffering is caused by clinging to illusory notions of identity and control, what is the escape from endless cycles of despair for those who self-injure? Eschewing emphasis on self-construction and management of oneself and one's environment, Buddhism moves in the opposite direction, toward letting go of the illusion of self and of control, instead looking outward toward the ubiquity of suffering. In this view, not only is self-injury not aberrant, it actually makes perfect sense. As demonstrated in chapters 2 and 7, within the lived contexts of those who self-injure, NSSI *works*.

If we as researchers are willing to open up our own restrictive definitions of NSSI, the discussion can move toward a much more activist position as we strive to reveal and remedy root causes of suffering around us, particularly— though not exclusively—among young people. To do this, however, we have to let go of some of our own clinging as researchers and practitioners. If we are too invested in narrow definitions, we will miss the connections to universal suffering, thus perpetuating the stigma of deviance associated with NSSI.

I have been guilty of this particular point as a chapter writer for this book, but I was lucky to be set straight by my student proofreader. In the first complete draft of my chapter, I carelessly referred to people who engage in NSSI as 'self-injurers,' thus reducing them to one socially disapproved behavior. My hubris as a tenured professor had blinded me to my own insensitivity so that I almost rhetorically dehumanized ("othered") the very people who I was trying to help.

We have seen throughout this book that researchers are generally satisfied that the reason people self-injure is to deal with feelings of anxiety, isolation, and so forth. But we can still dig further: What are the reasons why people who self-injure feel so stressed? Just taking adolescents as an example, we could investigate what social conditions lead to such levels of anxiety among these young people and what we can do to remedy the situation. And who could better answer this question than adolescents who engage in NSSI? A very different approach to NSSI could be toward encouraging people who self-injure to recognize the *value* of their experience in helping to expose and remedy social, economic, and cultural stressors needing immediate attention.

Validation of suffering is a form of compassion. It is comforting for both those who give it and those who receive it. "Compassion" is *feeling with*. Similarly, "communication" is *sharing with*. "Community" is *being with*. These words suggest a horizontal distribution of meaning, power and resources. We often use these words in our research, yet there is a tendency in scholarship—much like the medical industry—to perceive the world in a top-down fashion exemplified by the often denounced "medical model" (see, Kleinman 1988). By stressing the "witness" of compassion, we can turn our traditional expert/patient model around by recognizing and validating the wealth of expertise shared among people who self-injure. Instead of constructing people who self-injure as a class unto themselves, what if we communicate with them as people with specialized knowledge pertaining to human suffering? How can their knowledge and experience help us to target and remedy social problems leading to NSSI?

The witness of suffering is about recognizing connection with others. Brendan Kelly (2011) touches briefly upon this notion in his brief discussion of how Buddhist concept of *dukkha* (suffering) can be applied in Western therapeutic practices:

> Buddhist teachings about the inevitability of *dukkha* in human life . . . can be used to place the complex situation of the individual within a broader framework, and provide a pathway towards a more balanced understanding of how one might reasonably expect to live patiently in the world. The Buddhist perspective on dukkha guides people to take suffering less personally and may provide some relief for certain distressed individuals by helping them to re-frame their personal pain into a broader context.

Recognition that suffering is a normal human trait means tearing down walls built through perceptions of isolation. We have already seen the desire of many who engage in NSSI to construct communities via online communication (chapters 6 and 7). How can we as experts in our respective fields help build and maintain *positive, uplifting, mutually supportive*, and *compassionate* communities around the experience of suffering? (Unlike the brutal, destructive sort of community described in chapter 8!)

Although they don't mention Buddhism directly, Marta Carvahal and Nicole Parrish (chapter 1) stress the importance of "mindfulness" in working with patients. They define the term as focusing on the present moment—encouraging clients to be aware of their bodies, breath, and emotions. They go on to explain that people who self-injure often are unaware of their own motivations and that healthcare providers should be a source of compassion and knowledge.

Mindfulness is more than a short-term fix. It is a skill that one learns over time through practice. Thich Nhat Hanh (2014) writes that mindfulness begins with recognition of the body, including pain: "Our bodies often contain stress, pain, and suffering. Often, we ignore the body until the pain gets too great ... Sitting and breathing mindfully, we bring the mind back to the body and begin to recognize its presence and release the tension there" (67). And "Once we are calm, we can see more clearly. And when our vision is no longer clouded, we see with more understanding, and we naturally begin to feel compassion for ourselves and others. That is when true happiness becomes possible" (65). Looking inward, the mindful person finds connection with others.

Questioning one's own motivations is a crucial factor in being mindful. As we guide people who self-injure toward a mindful approach, we can encourage them to continually ask themselves the seemingly simple question, Why? We must never expect that we already know the reasons, but rather, we need to listen carefully. In this way, we who consider ourselves experts have much to learn about day-to-day struggles of people outside our institutional walls. Recalling the notion of impermanence, we need to approach the motivational causes of NSSI with our own beginners' minds, listening carefully, much like I had to listen to my proofreader about my careless use of words.

Furthermore, we need to always monitor *our own* motivations in communicating about NSSI. Why do we study NSSI? Why do we work with people who engage in NSSI? Ideally, our motives should be to relieve the suffering of others. It is possible, however, that when we make a career out of studying NSSI and/or working with people who engage in NSSI, our motives might be more about our own occupations, prestige, and reputation. Ideally, we can find ways to simultaneously improve the lives of others while furthering our careers, but compassion toward others must be our first objective. The rest will follow. This, of course, is consistent with that most famous of all Buddhist principles: karma.

Buddhism is a far more complex philosophy than anyone could summarize in a few pages. My goal in applying concepts of impermanence, suffering, mindfulness, and compassion to the ways in which we think about and practice communication pertaining to NSSI has not been to demonstrate mastery over the subject. Far from it! Rather, I have tried to apply the openness of my beginner's mind with respect to Buddhism toward Western approaches that seem unable to resolve self-injury as a social problem. I am suggesting that we loosen our grip on the definition that we cling to, consider the possible presence of self-serving professional motives pertaining to specialization and academic "turf," and think more widely about what repetitive, self-injurious behavior tells us about human suffering in all forms and settings.

I see value in the lived experience of people who self-injure, and I want them to know that their struggles are nothing more or less than manifestations of being human. Further, I want them to know that they have unique insight into building community among people everywhere through their own forms of communication in some ways that we scholars and clinicians are familiar with and in other ways that we have not yet imagined.

In writing these concluding thoughts, I am not suggesting that we stop treating or discussing NSSI entirely as we have been. Nor am I saying that we should consider people who self-injure as some form of resource to plunder in the hopes of improving the social order. Rather, as I think about the chapters in this book, I suggest that an effective path forward can be constructed through a more balanced approach than we typically consider in Western healthcare. Sometimes, the best course of action is to emphasize individual challenges, focusing on building belief in self-efficacy and agency via reinforcement of a positive sense of identity and a focused vision of what NSSI entails. But at the same time, we should also recognize that that perspective is not working very well when so many people are turning to NSSI as a secretive means of escape and relief and that the problem isn't going away.

Aaltola (2019) concludes her article by offering the suggestion that it's not a matter of discarding one form of thinking for another, but rather of blending them in ways that keep both paradigms in mind, sometimes putting stress here, sometimes there. The Western emphasis on fixed identity—whether of the self or, by extension, a concept such as NSSI—is appropriate, "as long as we remember that 'we' are constantly changing conceptual constellations, that our potency is always limited, and our words secondary in relation to somatic, experiential, and compassionate interconnectedness with the world and other beings" (247).

As we study how people communicate about, with, and through NSSI, it's important to remember that the words, thoughts, feelings, and behaviors that we associate with self-injury are imperfect constructs, but are nevertheless useful points of entry into suffering that occurs all around us. We need not limit our path toward better understanding and treatment by clinging too much to narrow definitions of what NSSI is, who engages in NSSI, or how it is done. Further, we—as researchers and scholars—and our friends, family members, colleagues, and neighbors who self-injure would all benefit from the mindfulness implied in a more horizontal approach toward sharing information about what NSSI is, what it means, and what we can do about it. In this way, we can better understand, discuss, and represent NSSI as more than stigmatized behavior practiced among some people, but rather, as a commonly chosen strategy of survival in a world full of pain, and ultimately, as a channel through which community can be strengthened, and suffering can be reduced.

NOTE

1. Buddhism is practiced among four different schools of thought, all sharing the same basic principles, but varying somewhat in practice: Zen, Mayahana, Theravada, and Vajrayana.

WORKS CITED

Aaltola, Elisa. "Confronting Suffering with Narrative Theory, Constructed Selfhood, and Control: Critical Perspectives by Simone Weil and Buddhist Metaphysics." *Journal of Disability and Religion* 23, no. 3 (2019): 227–250.

Bercholz, Samuel, and Sherab Chödzin Kohn, editors. *An Introduction to the Buddha and His Teachings.* New York: Barnes & Noble, Inc.

Dimeff, Linda, and Marsha M. Linehan. "Dialectical Behavior Therapy in a Nutshell." *The California Psychologist* 34 (2001): 10–13.

Jiang, Yongqiang, Jianing You, Xiaoling Zheng, and Min-Pei Lin. "The Qualities of Attachment with Significant Others and Self-Compassion Protect Adolescents from Non Suicidal Self-Injury." *School Psychology Quarterly* 32, no. 2 (2017): 143–155.

Kelley, Brendan D. "Self-Immolation, Suicide and Self-Harm in Buddhist and Western Traditions." *Transcultural Psychiatry* 48, no. 3 (2011): 299–317.

Kleinman, Arthur. *The Illness Narratives; Suffering, Healing, and the Human Condition.* New York: Basic Books, 1988.

Linehan, Marsha M. *Cognitive-Behavioral Treatment of Borderline Personality Disorder.* New York: The Guilford Press, 1993a.

Linehan, Marsha M. *Skills Training Manual for Treating Borderline Personality Disorder.* New York: The Guilford Press, 1993b.

Lopez, Donald S. "First There Is a Mountain (Then There Is No Mountain): How Science Brought Down the Buddha's Mount Meru." *Tricycle: The Buddhist Review* 18, no. 1. Accessed via https://tricycle.org/magazine-issue/fall-2008/, July 18, 2020.

Muehlenkamp, Jennifer J. "Empirically Supported Treatments and General Therapy Guidelines for Non-Suicidal Self-Injury." *Journal of Mental Health Counseling* 28, no. 2 (2006): 166–185.

Nhat Hahn, Thich. *How to Sit.* Berkeley, CA: Parallax Press, 2014.

Robins, Clive J. "Zen Principles and Mindfulness Practice in Dialectical Behavior Therapy." *Cognitive and Behavioral Practice* 9 (2002): 50–57.

Shapiro, Shauna L. (2009). "The Integration of Mindfulness and Psychology." *Journal of Clinical Psychology* 65, no. 6 (2009): 555–560.

Suzuki, Shunryu. *Zen Mind, Beginner's Mind.* New York: Weatherhill, 1970.

Thera, Nyanponika. "Seeing Things as They Are." In *The Vision of Dhamma: The Buddhist Writings of Nyanponika Thera*, edited by Bhikkhu Bodhi and York Beach. ME: Samuel Wiser, 1987. Reprinted in *An Introduction to the Buddha and His Teachings*, edited by Samuel Bercholz and Sherab Chödzin Kohn, 83–85. New York: Barnes & Noble, Inc.

Van Gelder, Kiera. *The Buddha and the Borderline: My Recovery from Borderline Personality Disorder Through Dialectical Behavior Therapy, Buddhism, and Online Dating.* Oakland, CA: New Harbinger Publications, Inc., 2010.

Index

adolescents: entertainment patterns, 183–85, 187–90; family relationships, xv, 57–75; popular conceptions about, xi, 102, 125; risk of self-injury, 17, 37, 52, 57, 87–90, 95–96, 99, 142, 162, 183–84, 194, 199
anger: ability to communicate, 10, 13, 64; as immediate precursor to self-injury, 95, 120–21, 124, 144, 147; occurrence in conjunction with self-injury, xi, 10, 59, 68; reduction of, 86, 156
anxiety, 4–7, 17, 27, 58–60, 72, 89, 147. *See also* stress
Autobiographical Self-Enhancement Training (ASET), 38–53

biological correlates, 10, 83–84, 122, 137
blame, 8, 126, 156, 197. *See also* self-criticism
boundary maintenance, 21, 27–28, 62, 65–72, 75, 85, 88, 166, 174
Buddhist philosophy, 193–203
bullying, 59, 84, 88, 125

catharsis, 114–15, 123, 125
chaotic circumstances: among families, 5–6, 194; in narrative analysis, 136, 143–49, 151, 155–57, 174, 177

coercion, xv, 62, 65–75, 101, 170
cognitive behavioral therapy, 12, 197
cognitive intervention, 38–39, 50
communication: between patients and healthcare providers, 3, 5, 11–14, 22–32, 137, 164–65, 167, 178; interpersonal, xiii, xv–xvi, 2–3, 5, 7, 11–14, 19–22, 59, 71–73, 84–91, 95–99, 102, 138, 161–68, 180; intrapersonal, xiii–xv, 1–3, 8, 13–14, 19, 22, 24, 85–86, 95, 102, 162–64, 168–70, 172–73, 177–79; nonsuicidal self-injury as, xii–xvi, 1–2, 5, 13–14, 20, 31, 87, 138, 161–63, 165, 177–80; nonverbal, xii, 114, 165. See also online forums; social communicative model
community: amid social media, xv; in *Fight Club*, xv, 161, 167–75; imagined, xv–xvi, 144, 150, 156; online, 113–18, 130, 135–36, 144, 154, 156–57, 188–89; re-establishment of, 200
compassion, 2, 7, 138, 196, 200–202
conflict: with authority figures, 143; in families and significant others, 2, 30, 58–59, 62, 64–74, 84, 87, 125, 156, 180; with friends, 87; in narrative analysis, 141, 155; as precursor to

self-injury, xv, 95, 98, 102, 125; reinforcing patterns, 89; with self, 177; strategies to deal with, 87, 98, 156, 162, 197
coping: as maladaptive strategy, 87, 165–67; and memories, 63; strategies and skills, xv, 7, 10, 68, 90, 95–96, 98–99, 113–15, 137, 139, 145, 147, 149,151, 156–57; as temporary relief, 3, 17, 64, 71, 74–75, 85
cultural discourse analysis (CuDA), 116–31
culture: among those who self-injure, xv, 116–19, 128–30; anthropological perspective, 135; as context for self-injury, xii, 1, 13, 84, 138, 156, 162, 200; dystopian culture, 167, 171, 176–77; popular culture, xvi, 114, 138, 164, 178; Western *vs.* Eastern culture, 197
cutting: discourse about, xii, xvi, 13, 29, 115, 120–24, 142–43, 144–46, 149–56, 188; and emotional regulation, 5–11, 13, 17–18, 128, 145, 147; as a form of self-injury, xi, 29, 37, 162–64, 173, 194, 197; measure of, 47; as self-punishment, 8–9, 11, 13, 144, 148, 156

depression: antidepressants, 5, 10; comorbidity with self-injury, xi, 4, 17, 60, 63, 72, 84, 88–89, 124, 149; reduction, xiv, 39; symptoms, 5, 39, 44, 58; reduction, 9, 45–48, 50–51, 54
Diagnostic and Statistical Manual of Mental Disorders, 57, 61, 75, 137
dialectical behavioral therapy (DBT), xiv, 11–13, 126, 195
diaries. *See* journaling
disabilities, 9, 113, 114, 177, 195, 198
disclosure, 90–91, 98, 114
dissociation, 3–5, 84, 96, 146–48, 161–62, 164–80
distress. *See* stress

emotional mind, 10–12
emotional regulation: self-injury as, xi, 5–8, 19–23, 39, 58, 62–63, 75, 84–87, 91, 115, 119–26, 129, 131, 138, 146–47, 149, 151, 154, 162, 166, 170, 172–73; therapeutic strategies for, xiv, 2–4, 7, 10–13, 21–28, 30–32, 40–43, 50–53, 68, 71, 94–97, 194–95, 201. See also catharsis
empathy, xv, 5, 29, 31–32, 58–59, 62, 65–70, 73, 113, 129
empowerment, xvi–xvii, 22, 25–26, 28, 31, 138, 197
environmental factors, 1–2, 20–21, 73, 87–90, 92, 98, 102, 115, 149, 165, 170, 172, 179, 197, 199
exercise, 24, 68
expressive writing, 38, 47

family dynamics: family history, 2; family involvement in therapy, 7–8; maladaptive family conditioning, 13, 57–59, 64, 71–72, 84; measurement of, 64; positive family support, 58, 68, 74–75, 88–90, 199, 202; as a precipitating condition of self-injury, xi–xv, 13, 62, 95, 97, 99, 120, 126, 136–37, 142, 144–45, 147, 154, 194; sibling relationships, xv, 58–75, 142, 194
Fight Club, xvi, 161–80, 200
friendship, xiv–xv, 42–43, 64, 71, 73, 84, 88, 90, 95, 97, 99, 121, 126, 137, 142, 145, 154, 156, 163, 179, 194–95, 199, 202
functions of NSSI: assessment of, 11, 13, 18–20, 30–31, 61, 101; communication of needs, 2; community-based, xv; controlling dissociative episodes, 3–4, 129; deterrent, 124; interpersonal, xv, 19–20, 27, 86, 88, 96, 115, 162–63, 174, 194; intrapersonal, 5–8, 19, 25–26, 86, 94–96, 115, 129, 163, 177, 194; narrative functions, 138, 144, 147–

48, 155, 158; socio-communicative functions, xv, 83–103, 117. *See also* coping; emotional regulation; self-punishment

gender, 6, 43, 51, 74, 141, 142, 162, 163, 176. See also masculinity
genetic factors, 73, 88
guilt, 1, 3, 9, 21, 59, 63, 126–27, 135, 148, 156, 198, 199. See also self-criticism

histories. *See* patient histories
hopefulness, 27, 12, 32, 135–36, 138–39, 150–51, 153, 156
hopelessness, 51, 84, 125, 139

identity, 4, 12, 72, 141, 146, 163, 167, 171–74, 176, 180, 195, 197, 199, 202
internalization, 58, 61, 66–68, 70, 72–73, 83, 173, 177, 179
International Society for the Study of Self-Injury, xiv, 1
interpretive research methodology, 135–36. *See also* cultural discourse analysis
isolation, xi, xvi, 84, 96–97, 101, 126, 130, 145, 167, 179, 198–200

journaling, xiv–xv, 37–53, 92, 97–98, 197

listening, 42, 121, 129, 135–36, 157

masculinity, 163, 165, 167–69, 176–77, 180
media representations of NSSI, xi–xii, xvi, 138, 161–80, 183–84, 194
medical model, 137–39, 148–49, 200
medication, 5, 9, 11, 40, 44, 167
micro-longitudinal designs, 85, 91–103
mindfulness, 2, 7, 10, 12–14, 24, 195–96, 200–202

narrative: emancipatory power of, 114, 137–38, 195; fictional narrative analysis, xvi, 164–80; illness narratives, xv, 136–39; narrative analysis methodology, 135–41; online narratives, 141–58; potential harms, 114
negative thoughts, 3, 7–8, 123
nonsuicidal self-injury (NSSI): defined, xi, 1, 37, 57, 162, 183, 198; motivations for, xv, 1–8, 13–14, 23, 24, 30, 139, 168, 170, 171, 201; precipitants, xv, 85, 88, 91, 96–98, 100, 117, 119–22, 125, 127, 130–31; prevalence, 17–18, 37, 50, 57–58, 183; reduction, xiv–xv, 37–52, 91. *See also* cutting, functions of NSSI

online forums: etiquette, 115; harmful content, 114; recruitment in research, 39–40; Reddit, xv, 39, 135–36, 141–42, 144, 151, 154–56; r/selfharm, xv, 135–39, 142–58; *Sharp Talk*, 115–16; SuicideForum.com, xv, 118–31

pain: emotional, 3, 6–7, 12, 63, 123–26, 128–29, 131, 138, 164, 168, 173, 198, 200, 203; endurance, 38–39; physical, 3, 6, 12, 19, 37–39, 63, 83, 123–24, 127–30, 138, 144, 146–47, 150, 161–62, 164–69, 173–78, 201, 203; processing, 83
patient histories, 2, 7–8, 10, 18, 38, 44, 46, 50, 52, 57, 83, 89, 91, 97–99, 102, 118, 144
peer influence, 59, 64, 71, 84, 88–90, 95, 98–99, 118. See also online forums
position, 25–28
precipitants, 15, 85, 88, 91, 95–99, 117, 119–22, 125, 127, 131

radical acceptance, 12
recovery, xiv, 22–24, 27, 68, 114, 131, 148–49, 152, 155
rejection, 14, 29, 84–85, 88–89, 95–98, 102, 116, 176, 198

scars: acceptance of, xii, xvi, 5, 150, 173; healed, 146; hidden, 5, 142–43, 145; as representation, 7, 126, 130–31, 138, 147, 149, 151; socially sanctioned, xi
secrecy, 5, 18, 40, 90, 148, 157, 168, 202
self-awareness, 2, 13, 23
self-criticism, xiv, 37–39, 44–48, 50–52, 84, 95, 114
self-harm. *See* non-suicidal self-injury
self-punishment, 3, 8–9, 96, 128, 147–49, 153, 162
self-regulatory approach (SRA), 18–32
self-worth, 38–39, 95, 113, 127–28
social communicative model, 84–92, 94–99, 102–3, 172
stigma, xiii, xv–xvi, 37, 40, 59, 85–86, 90, 113–14, 130, 136, 148, 156, 195, 198–99, 203
storytelling. *See* narrative
stress, xi, 2–3, 5–7, 10–12, 17, 19, 25, 39, 59, 64, 68, 71, 74, 83–89, 95–100, 115–16, 119–23, 126–27, 137, 149–50, 154, 156–57, 162, 173, 194, 198–202. See also anxiety
Structural-Process Model (SPM), 21–32
suicide: association with non-suicidal self-injury, 57, 63, 68, 113–14, 129, 175; non-suicidal self-injury as deterrent to suicide, 26, 124; suicidal behaviors, 102; suicidal discursive patterns, xv, 117–18, 119, 164; suicidal ideation, xiv, 27, 37–39, 44–51, 57, 100, 102, 124
symptom constellations, 17–18

therapeutic approaches, 2–14, 18–32, 37, 64, 126, 131, 164, 194–95, 197, 200. See also dialectical behavioral therapy (DBT)
trauma, 2, 4, 7–8, 10–12, 17–18, 20, 24, 30, 84, 166
triggering, 5, 52, 59, 84, 88, 96, 118–19, 120, 122, 126, 129, 139, 163, 166, 175–76, 178

wise mind, 10–12

About the Authors

Mike Alvarez, PhD, is a postdoctoral diversity and innovation scholar in the Department of Communication at the University of New Hampshire. He received his doctorate from the University of Massachusetts Amherst, where he taught courses in film and media studies, television production, human communication and technology, forensics, and thanatology. He is a recipient of the Paul and Daisy Soros Fellowship and author of the forthcoming book, *The Paradox of Suicide and Creativity*. Visit him at mfalvarez.net or follow him on Twitter @mfalvarez121.

Lisann Anders, PhD, is a teaching and research assistant at the University of Zurich, Switzerland. She earned her doctorate from the University of Zurich. Her book *Communication in Postmodern Urban Fiction: The Shadow of Imagination* discusses communicative strategies in postmodern urban American fiction. Other research interests include Shakespeare as well as literature in conjunction with popular culture in the form of adaptations. Previous publications include "Making Her Own Destiny: Disney's Diverse Females" in *4th Wave Feminism in Science Fiction and Fantasy* and "The Normal Abnormal: Identity Formation in the Circus Space" in *The Big Top on the Big Screen: Explorations of the Circus in Film*. Her current project is an edited volume on the comic book and Netflix series *Umbrella Academy*.

Warren J. Bareiss, PhD, studies relationships among communication and culture, with an emphasis on health, at the University of South Carolina Upstate. He earned his doctorate from Indiana University and his master's from the Annenberg School for Communication at the University of Pennsylvania. He earned a postdoctoral graduate certificate in health communication from the Arnold School for Public Health and the School of Journalism at the

University of South Carolina. Dr. Bareiss' research has been published in *The Journal of Medical Humanities* and *Health: An Interdisciplinary Journal for the Social Study of Health, Illness and Medicine*, and other journals and books. Subjects that he teaches include health narrative, communication research methods, and health communication messaging. Dr. Bareiss also developed and coordinates the health communication minor at USC Upstate.

Marta Carvalhal, LISW-CP, is a licensed independent social worker who has been practicing in outpatient and inpatient behavioral settings for over fifteen years. She has also worked in the psychiatric ward of the emergency department. In addition, she is an instructor for the College of Social Work at the University of South Carolina. She combines her enthusiasm and energy with her experience and evidence-based research treatment to deliver the best for her patients.

Kathryn Fox, PhD, received her doctorate in clinical psychology from Harvard in 2019. She is currently an assistant professor at the University of Denver in the Department of Psychology. Her research takes a multi-method approach to better understand risk for and to increase accessibility to treatment and prevention programs for suicide and self-harming behaviors.

Carolyn Helps is a graduate student in the Clinical Lifespan Psychology program at the University of Victoria in British Columbia, Canada. Her research seeks to understand how individuals are able to manage, reduce, or cease engaging in self-damaging behaviors, and how this subsequently affects mental health and wellbeing. Carolyn previously earned her Bachelor of Arts (Hons.) in Psychology at the University of Victoria.

Jill M. Hooley, DPhil, is a professor of psychology in the Department of Psychology at Harvard University. She is also head of the Experimental Psychopathology/Clinical Psychology Program at Harvard. Dr. Hooley received her doctorate from Oxford University. She has received grants from the NIMH and the Borderline Personality Disorder Research Foundation and published many journal articles and book chapters on a broad range of topics. Together with Jim Butcher and Matthew Nock, she is also the author of the textbook, *Abnormal Psychology*. Dr. Hooley received the A. T. Beck Award for Excellence in Psychopathology Research in 2000 and in 2015 she was the recipient of the Joseph Zubin Award for Lifetime Achievement in Psychopathology Research from the Society for Research in Psychopathology.

Tina In-Albon, PhD, is a professor for clinical child and adolescent psychology and psychotherapy at the University of Koblenz-Landau, Landau, Germany. She is also head of the Landauer outpatient clinic for children and adolescent psychotherapy. Her research focuses on non-suicidal self-injury and anxiety disorders.

Anita Kwashie is a clinical science PhD student at the University of Minnesota. Her research concerns cognitive deficits in severe psychopathology and their relationship to behavioral and clinical outcomes.

John Levitt, PhD, FAED, FIAEDP, CEDS-S, has more than forty years' experience in working with clients who suffer from self-harm, eating disorders, and symptoms related to histories of trauma and abuse; he has also been instrumental in developing practice-based models of treatment for those populations. He has taught classes on psychological and emotional trauma at the graduate level and consults with other clinicians on clinical treatment challenges. He has been an active participant in the fields of eating disorders, family therapy, self-harm, and trauma as a clinician, consultant, program developer, supervisor/trainer, and presenter. Dr. Levitt has been clinical director of more than five treatment programs and has worked in hospital-based programs and private practice. He has taught widely, coauthored one book, coedited three other books, and has over eighty articles and publications. Dr. Levitt has emphasized the importance of "giving back" to the community and has provided over 200 pro bono workshops. He is noted for his exciting and useful trainings and publications on how to successfully facilitate client change using the therapeutic relationship—for even the most symptomatically challenging client. Dr. Levitt currently maintains a private practice in the Northwest suburbs of Chicago.

Shuang Liu, PhD, is an assistant professor of communication at University of South Carolina Upstate. She earned her doctorate in communication from Washington State University. Her research is focused on learning about how media, especially new media technologies, improve health and how such information is processed and understood. Her work can be found in *Journal of Health Communication, Computers in Human Behavior*, and so forth.

Janine Lüdtke, PhD, is a licensed psychotherapist and works in an inpatient psychiatric unit for children and adolescents. Her research focuses on non-suicidal self-injury

Yanni Ma, PhD, is an assistant professor in the Department of Speech Communication at Oregon State University. Her research centers on science, environment, and risk communication. Specifically, she is interested in understanding the underlying mechanism of people processing persuasive messages and what contributes to the effectiveness and ineffectiveness of those messages.

Nicole S. Parrish, MD, is a medical doctor who completed her adult psychiatry residency training at Prisma Health/University of South Carolina. She is currently completing fellowship training in child and adolescent psychiatry at the Virginia Treatment Center for Children/VCU Health. Prior to becoming a medical doctor, she worked in the Virginia public school system as an integrated classroom teacher and continues to be passionate about education and the impact mental illness has on every aspect of a child's life.

Marc Schmid, PhD, is a leading psychologist at the Department of Adolescent Psychiatry, University Psychiatric Clinics Basel in Switzerland where he also is a lecturer in psychology and head of Child and Adolescent Liaison Services. He has been teaching cognitive behavioral therapy since 2009.

Taru Tschan, PhD, is an advanced doctoral student and in training to become a psychotherapist. Her research focuses on non-suicidal self-injury and familial relationships.

Brianna J. Turner, PhD, RPsych, is an assistant professor in clinical psychology at the University of Victoria, where she directs the Risky Behaviour Lab. Dr. Turner's research focuses on understanding when and why people engage in behaviors that are physically harmful to themselves, including non-suicidal self-injury, suicidal behaviors, and disordered eating. Her current research uses micro-longitudinal and longitudinal methods to observe how these behaviors change over minutes, hours, days, months, and years. In addition, her research uses epidemiological surveys to understand the population-level health impact of these behaviors across the lifespan. Dr. Turner's research has been funded by the Canadian Institutes of Health Research, the Michael Smith Foundation for Health Research, the SickKids Foundation, and the Social Sciences and Humanities Research Council.

Shirley Wang (A.M., Harvard University) is a PhD candidate in clinical psychology with a secondary in computational science and engineering at Harvard University. She works with Dr. Matthew Nock and is funded by the National Science Foundation Graduate Research Fellowship Program. Shirley's research aims to improve the understanding of why people engage in behaviors that are harmful to themselves, including eating disorder behaviors, self-injury, and suicide. She is particularly interested in using mathematical and computational modeling to formalize theories in psychopathology.

www.ingramcontent.com/pod-product-compliance
Lightning Source LLC
Chambersburg PA
CBHW050904300426
44111CB00010B/1370